Inner Transformations Using Essential Oils

Powerful Cleansing Protocols for
Increased Energy and More Radiant Health

Inner Transformations Using Essential Oils: Powerful Cleansing Protocols for Increased Energy and More Radiant Health is not intended as medical advice. It is not provided to diagnose, prescribe, or treat any condition of the body. The information in this book should not be used as a substitute for medical counseling with a health professional. Neither the author nor the publisher accepts responsibility for such use.

The opinions and ideas expressed in this book are uniquely the authors and neither Life Science Publishing nor Young Living have anything to do with the information in this book even though the majority of the products mentioned in this book are from Young Living Essential Oils.

ISBN #978-0-9894997-9-8

Printed in the United States of America

Life Science Publishing
Orem UT 84605
www.LifeSciencePublishers.com

800.336.6308

Inner Transformations Using Essential Oils

Powerful Cleansing Protocols for
Increased Energy and More Radiant Health

Dr. LeAnne Deardeuff, DC & Dr. David Deardeuff, DC

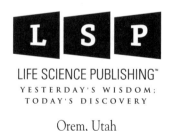

LIFE SCIENCE PUBLISHING™
YESTERDAY'S WISDOM:
TODAY'S DISCOVERY

Orem, Utah

This book is dedicated to:

Infant Palmer
And **All Your Cousins**

*This, my life's work, is to assist you
in having a healthier life than I did.*

This is also dedicated to your
Grandfather *who without his help,
it would never have come to be.*

ACKNOWLEDGMENTS

I owe a tremendous amount of thanks to my husband, David Deardeuff, D.C. who has had to put up with years of lupus from me. I thank him for staying with me. I thank him for assisting me in my quest for health. I thank him for putting up with all my diet changes and supplements and doctor searches. I thank him for his research and ideas. In addition, especially I thank him for reading my thoughts, listening to my voice and writing them out for me so you can listen also. Without him, this book would still be stuck in my head.

Also a great a big thanks to my daughter-in-law, Bethany, who showed up for me and giving me the clue about MTHFR syndrome which has made a tremendous shift in my health. I pray that you too can now receive help and health. A huge thanks goes to her husband, Michael, who had to feed children and take care of his home as well as work a job as we went through this healing journey and crisis. I love you, Michael.

Large applauds and thanks go to another daughter-in-law, Mindy, who had amazing ideas for the cover and to Paul Springer who always brings thoughts to light! What a talent. I especially am grateful for his dropping everything to do it! It is beautiful. Thank you so much.

And to my readers and clients, thank you for applauding me and keeping me going. I am grateful for your questions, which assisted me in moving forward with this revision, allowing me to see what needed to be changed.

I appreciate my best friends putting up with my grumpiness while I write, having dyslexia and dysgraphia has its own challenges to be able to pull things out of my head and put it on paper. So grateful for voice memos on my phone and a microphone and digital recorder that can record thoughts and a great transcriber, Lori Bruton who listened to all the craziness in my head, yet still got it on paper and edited the chaos to make sense.

Thank you to Sarah, my daughter, who stayed up "early" to read the first edition of "Inner Transformations" aloud into a recorder when we discovered that our manuscript of the first book was missing! Well, it was a great health class for her I am sure!

Thank you to a great VA, Debbie Twomey, who took over my blogs and newsletters, while she was ill and I was writing. That was indeed a great blessing for everyone!

And a star-studded song of thanks to Dr. Mary Starr Carter, D.C. for the great forward to the book!!

I appreciate you all,
Dr. LeAnne

TABLE OF CONTENTS

FOREWORD

I remember the first patient I had in 2004 who needed Dr. LeAnne's Cleansing Protocols. He was a young man in his 30's who had terrible painful cysts under his arms, on his neck and every warm area of the body. Even walking was painful for him most days. Before he got to my office he had traveled all over the world seeing doctors and finally had the cystic skin surgically removed and grafted cyst free skin from his thighs on his underarms and inner thighs. It worked for a little bit but the cysts still came back. When I took his health history I found out that he didn't have regular bowel movements. In fact it was quite "normal" for him to go 10 days between bowel movements.... My mouth dropped and I proceeded to tell him that those toxins accumulating in his body had to get out somehow and they were getting out through his skin and that was why he was having such bad acne cysts. "No doctor told you this? " I asked. "No", he said.

I proceeded to apply essential oils to his spine and immediately a terrible smell rose out from his back proving my theory that his body was toxic and the only way his system could get rid of it was through the skin. I did my best to coach him through cleansing but my knowledge was limited then and I fumbled my way through it. I saw more clients through the years that needed cleansing protocols but I just couldn't find the right resources until Dr. LeAnne printed her book in 2006.

Inner Transformations Using Essential Oils: Power Cleansing Protocols for Increased Energy and Better Health was BRILLANT. Unlike so many cleansing books out there this gave specifics of why we needed cleansing, the difference between different cleanses, and exactly how to cleanse. She took out all the guesswork and saved me countless hours coaching my patients. I kept her books for sale in the office and our patients got better faster because they had this simple useful tool they could start using right away.

A few years after I started sharing her books I got the opportunity to meet her in person at a business training. She was funny, kind, generous, loved God and had a pure heart for helping others. Her experience working with thousands of patients was impressive but I think it's her own personal experiences that make her a fabulous doctor. Her family of 12 children and 8 grandchildren so far and her own personal health struggles are what make LeAnne one of the most real and down to earth doctors I know.

Her husband David Deardeuff was also a Chiropractor working by her side. He was the technical genius behind this book, spending countless hours in research and pulling the clinical experiences together.

In 2010, I would find her book and teachings even more powerful in my own life as I started having children. Unfortunately, in 2011 I had two miscarriages and decided I needed to re-visit her Cleansing Protocols and teachings. I did and I believe the birth of my beautiful baby girl Sarah Grace in April of 2013 is a direct result of the Cleansing Protocols I followed and Dr. LeAnne's teachings.

Inner Transformations using Essential Oils will be unlike any book you have read before on cleansing. Its layout and protocols are perfect for all readers. Moreover, since cleansing is the foundation of optimal health most everyone will find information that they need. Whether you are struggling with a serious digestive disorder, trying to get pregnant, struggling with hormonal issues, or suffer with bad skin issues there is information in this book that you need.

I can say from both a professional and personal level that the readers of this book will find the information extremely helpful on their health journey, but for me **"Inner Transformations Using Essential oils"** has changed my life.

God Bless your Health Journey;

Mary Starr Carter
the Total Wellness Doc and Mom
www.thetotalwellnessdoc.com
Young Living Diamond Star Distributor

PREFACE

"Inner Transformations" has needed an update from the day it came out in print at the 2006 convention in Salt Lake City. On that day many of the supplements changed or their names changed and new supplements came out. I wonder what will happen this year!

I also knew that I hadn't completed the chapter on metals. That I was missing information on the small intestine nor did I have information about male hormones!

Little did I know that our whole world would be rocked a few years later with the introduction of Progessence Plus! What a miracle that has been for so many women! I had to rewrite the women's hormone chapter and had so much more information it turned into a booklet!

Every year I knew I needed to rewrite the book. And every year I procrastinated. This year, I started a group on Facebook, called The Cleansing Club with "Inner Transformations Using Essential Oils". There were so many questions about the Protocol of Colon Cleansing since the products names had changed; that I decided it was time for a revision.

Therefore, readers out there, pay attention when the products change and write a note in the cover of the book so you can remember! It took me 8 years to revise this one!!

Dr. LeAnne

INTRODUCTION

I became interested in natural healing in 1988 after years of migraine headaches, chronic fatigue and allergies. I was strictly a Western allopathic medicine person until then. After I had lain in bed for most of the time during a three year stretch, the medical profession finally told me that my problem was psychological; that I didn't like to do housework so I was bringing this problem on myself. They recommended to my husband that he divorce me because I was "lazy."

About that time Cheryl, a long lost friend of mine, called me and I told her about my health problems. She told me that she had suffered from similar problems and was using herbs and a special diet to clean up a yeast infection. She suggested that I go with her to her doctor to get some help. Her doctor was a retired medical surgeon in Maryland where we lived who had left the medical field after discovering that the organs he was removing were covered in a white coating. Upon investigation he found that they were covered in *candida albicans*, commonly called yeast. He had decided to go into natural healing to teach people how to recover from yeast infections and also how to prevent it from destroying their bodies. I learned a great deal about colon cleansing and herbal treatments from him.

Cheryl and I started taking a class taught by Caroline Tubman. She was a Nature's Sunshine distributor and was a certified teacher for Doctor John Christopher's Academy of Herbal Health. We took several weekend classes from her on herbs and natural healing. We watched hours of Dr. Christopher's video tapes. One of the things that he strongly believed was that "death begins in the colon." He believed that 95% of all diseases could be cleared up by getting the colon healthy. He also talked at length about how herbs worked. He explained that the active ingredients of herbs were in the oils of the plant. He taught that the best way to use or assimilate an herb was either in a tea that steeped the oil out of the herb into the water or in a tincture that drew the oil out into the alcohol. This was my first awareness of such a thing as an essential oil.

I was first introduced to essential oils themselves later in 1988. I was at a health food store and saw an advertisement for a miracle cure called tea tree oil. I bought a large $4.00 bottle of it and took it home to see if it would indeed cure my skin fungus infections or my yeast problems. After using it for about a month with absolutely no results, I was convinced that essential oils were another hoax from the health food industry. I was determined I wouldn't ever waste my money on something like that again. Later I learned that the quality and purity of an essential oil have everything to do with its effectiveness. Obviously the product I bought was not the best.

I had a friend who tried to sell me on Melaleuca brand tree tea oil for about 5 years but, scarred by earlier experiences, I resisted. Finally in 1996, she convinced me to use her oil for a few of my problems. Finally, here was an oil that delivered on its claims. About a year later, a dear friend introduced me to Young Living Essential Oils and I was hooked. I started using the oils in my chiropractic practice to loosen tight muscles. Just a drop or two of the Release essential oil blend on tight muscles gave me instant results. My patients' muscles relaxed and I was able to adjust them with a lot less effort.

I read everything I could get my hands on about essential oils. I listened to tapes and went to seminars and trainings. But the best education I received was trying the oils out on myself, friends, family and patients. I tried them all and learned what they did firsthand.

It wasn't until I started using essential oils full time instead of herbal remedies that I finally got control of my chronic fatigue. I started recommending Young Living Essential Oils to my patients for various other complaints such as fibromyalgia and infertility. We used it for scoliosis and for emotional upsets and everything in between. The results were often phenomenal. Happy patients referred their friends to me in droves and as I helped them I learned even more.

Through this book I hope to help many people overcome chronic problems that have been plaguing them too long. My hope is that my experience using essential oils and other natural remedies—for the diseases I have personally overcome or helped my patients overcome—will enable many more people to enjoy better health as they apply the principles that are taught herein.

How to use this book:

After discussing the hows and whys of using essential oils, I begin with information on how to cleanse the colon, as it is the major eliminator of toxins in the body and must be cleaned first before any other cleanse can be fully effective. The best time of year to clean the colon according to Chinese acupuncture is the fall, followed by the urinary tract in the winter, the gall bladder and liver in the spring, the heart and small intestine in the early summer, the stomach and spleen in the late summer, and the lungs and colon in the fall again. It would be ideal to just routinely follow this schedule year after year. However, if you have never done a cleanse, start with the colon no matter what time of the year it is! Cleansing is probably the most important thing you can do for your health, and the colon comes first, because if your elimination system has nowhere to dump its toxins, you could become quite ill when cleansing. Good health to you and happy cleansing.

— Dr. Leanne Deardeuff, DC
　Radiant Life Healing Center
　Lehi, Utah

CHAPTER 1

Is Your Body Toxic?

What is going on in the world today? Childhood obesity is rampant. Sugar diabetes Type II is on a rapid rise. Chronic fatigue, fibromyalgia, allergies, and other nutrition-related diseases are common. Cancer in all its manifestations stalks the land, accompanied by dreaded forms of treatment. It seems that everyone is on some type of prescription drug, and so are their friends. Surgery is commonplace to remove diseased or dysfunctional organs. In short, we are afflicted by diseases and "cures" of all kinds that our parents and grandparents never even heard of. Why is that? What can we do about it?

How did we get in this mess?

Our current culture and lifestyle is one of "busy"ness and hurriedness. We have too many things to do. We are running from one place to another, this meeting or that meeting, this event or that—our own or our children's. Because we are so busy we demand convenience. Convenience stores within gas stations thrive because that means one less stop on the way home to get something that we need. Walmart and the like are successful because we can make one stop and get everything we need in one place. That means less running around! Cell phones are a must. We can make our calls while on the run now instead of having to wait until we get home.

Unfortunately, this culture/lifestyle also means that fast food is becoming our main diet instead of a treat once in a while. Cookbooks have changed drastically over the years. Instead of recipes calling for basic ingredients, the cookbooks say to put in a box of this mix or a bottle of that prepared sauce, etc. We don't have time to enjoy our own vegetables that are organically grown, free from pesticides, herbicides and synthetic fertilizers. Our foods often come packaged in plastics; they are filled with colorings and preservatives to make them look better and to extend their shelf life. The highly-processed food that we eat typically is dead and laced with chemicals. The cleaners and soaps that we use are full of materials that are toxic to our bodies. Even a lot of the supplements we take to try to compensate for nutritionally-depleted foods are synthetic and of no use to us. We have traded our health for convenience, to keep up with the pace of modern life.

Reductionist vs. Wholistic

Increasingly we find we must turn to medicine for help (or so we believe), but a moment's thought will show that Western medicine is not up to the task. What we always hear called "health care" is really just "illness care." It doesn't keep us healthy, as evidenced by the increasing prevalence of disease and poor health among us. Instead we find that modern Western medical care is focused on "fixing" or hiding symptoms rather than setting us on the correct path to health. We might ask ourselves, If our health care system were truly effective, would we need to keep building these huge hospitals, mighty monuments to medicine?

Modern Western medicine rather consistently looks at the part instead of the whole, seeking always to reduce things to their smallest constituents. Doctors look at each organ and each disease state in isolation. If a drug doesn't make it stop bothering us, surgery might be next.

But the human body is a marvelous, complex organism designed to function as a whole; it's not just a collection of parts. For that matter, it is also meant to function as part of the whole of life; we will discuss our host relationship with microorganisms in Chapter 5. Living beings can better be healed with life-giving things than with drugs. But we are in the grip of a philosophy that is anti-life, as antibiotics are seen as conferring healthful benefits. Ironically, as microorganisms become more and more resistant to *anti*biotics, we may find we have to turn at last to *pro*biotics, life-supporting bacteria rather than life-killing drugs.

And what about our crazy situation with prescription drugs?! These are often developed as pharmaceutical chemists ask "What is the active ingredient in this medicinal plant that makes it work? How can we isolate that ingredient and make it synthetically so we can patent it and earn money from it?" The other minerals and enzymes and co-agents in the plant are ignored, yet in nature these constituents act synergistically to help the herb work at its best. When you take away all the other parts of the herb and use only its so-called active ingredient it becomes unnatural and creates unwanted side affects.

Generally speaking, whole foods, herbs and oils do not have such side effects. An example of this is apple seeds. How many times has someone eaten an apple seed by accident and not gotten ill? Yet reductionist science would cry out that apple seeds contain *prunasin* which releases cyanide when ingested. Cyanide is a known poison! But the other elements in the seed keep it from being poisonous to our systems.

Looking at physiology, it is interesting to see that the chemicals that keep the body going are <u>complete</u> vitamins and minerals. The best way, if not the only way, to get vitamins and minerals into our bodies is to eat the plants that God, or Nature if you prefer, has prepared for our use.

On the other hand, the drugs and synthetic vitamins that we take are actually foreign to the body! Dr. Carl Pfieffer, a well-known medical doctor from Naperville, Illinois, did a lot of work with people who had mental illnesses. He found that chronic depression is caused by a chemical imbalance in the brain and that the missing chemicals are vitamins and minerals. He used megadoses of vitamins to heal his patients' problems.

Synthetic vs. Natural Vitamins

But even vitamins and minerals get tampered with. Natural vitamins have been studied to see what their "active ingredient" is and how to make it synthetically, thus making more profit from selling it. An example is vitamin C. Most vitamin C sold over-the-counter is actually ascorbic acid. In fact vitamin C is often defined as ascorbic acid, but ascorbic acid is really only the outer part of the natural vitamin C molecule, an anti-oxidant that protects the rest of the compound. Most manufacturers do not include the citrus bioflavonoids and various other components that contribute importantly to the full range of activity of true vitamin C. Vitamins created within whole foods will have all of their coagents and will work with the body, while so-called vitamins that are made synthetically or have only some of their parts may actually be toxic. Further, a study by University of California researchers found that people who consumed 500 Mg of ascorbic acid daily had a 2.5 times higher rate of hardening of the arteries. The discoverer of vitamin C, Dr. Albert Szent-Georgi, at first believed that vitamin C was simply ascorbic acid, and the vitamin industry quotes him to this effect, but he later found that ascorbic acid alone did not have the benefits of the true vitamin C molecule.

Some Toxins Just Don't Leave

What does the body do with toxins that we ingest in so many ways? Because it cannot recognize them as natural substances it doesn't know how to deal with many of them. Although some simple substances may be excreted by the kidney, larger unnatural chemicals cannot be. Since the body can't metabolize them in the liver, it has to store them in the tissues to keep them from circulating and doing harm. Usually it will encase the toxin in a fat molecule and store it in the skin or in the brown fat surrounding the organs. The liver also stores a lot of toxins itself, which impairs its ability to function optimally. These toxins actually cause liver damage. Toxins also create free radicals which attack and damage cells throughout the body, and are a known cause of cancer.

One of the most common types of cancer in the United States is colorectal cancer, which means cancer of the colon or the rectum located at the distal end of the colon. For 2005, the estimated number of new cases of colorectal cancer in the U.S. Alone was over 153,000.

Colorectal cancers can be attributed chiefly to constipation, resulting from two main factors: lack of fiber in the diet and dehydration stemming from insufficient ingestion of water. For years the American Medical Association has been trying to get people to eat more fiber in their diets to help combat colon cancer. Bran was once all the rage, then oats. The truth of the matter is, if we were eating a more natural diet full of both cooked and raw fruits and vegetables and whole grains, and especially fermented foods and fermentable fiber, not only would we have adequate fiber in our diets but also more enzymes to help the body digest the foods that we eat, and more vitamins and minerals to keep us healthy.

From Wheat to Nutritionless Starch

White flour is a perfect example of how the food we eat has been stripped of its fiber, enzymes and nutrients. Looking at the whole grain, the bran is the outside layer. It is full of fiber and minerals. Inside the bran is the endosperm. The endosperm is made up of mostly starch that will feed the plant as it grows.

The germ is in the center of the grain. It is the life of the seed. It houses the hormones, fatty acids, vitamins and other micronutrients necessary to help the plant germinate and grow. It can be considered the life of the seed or grain. But during the processing of the white flour, the bits of brown bran or fiber are sifted out, the germ is removed to keep the flour from becoming rancid and then the flour is bleached to be a beautiful white color instead of brown or yellow. But what is left is nutritionless starch. This nutritionless starch is then "enriched" by having spraying synthetic vitamins and minerals sprayed back onto it, but we have already discussed how these synthetic vitamins are foreign to the body. The original wheat is further abused in the process of being turned into various supermarket products. But wheat (along with other grains) is an essential part of our diets and has been for millenia. Please see the blog on my website titled Wheat – the Good and Bad of It at http://doctorleanne.com/wheat/

White flour, so common in our diet, when mixed with water (or dairy products), produces a type of glue. To demonstrate this, just think back to your childhood to the recipe for paper mache paste (white flour and water) or glue substitute (white flour and milk) you may have used in school. Real old-timers remember when it was common to use white flour and water as wallpaper paste. It worked well and lasted a long, long time.

This same gluey substance, made from white flour products combined with dairy products and/or mucus, makes a coating on the inside of the bowel, blocking the mucous glands and the peristaltic action of the colon. Dr. Bernard Jensen calls this the "lining" of the bowel;

All this adds up to what is commonly called the Standard American Diet (SAD), of which the foundation is the "four deadly whites": White flour, white sugar, processed milk, and too much salt, in foods that have been stripped of vitamins, minerals and enzymes. Other elements of the SAD diet include an excess of chemical additives and a deficiency of fruit, vegetables and fiber.

Why Cleanse?

Why cleanse? In short, to rid ourselves of the effects of our SAD diet that creates a clogged digestive tract. With 70-80 percent of the immune system in the digestive tract, it is obvious that we must have our digestive tracts in top condition to ward off illness. Also, a clogged or sluggish digestive tract obviously means less nutrition for the body. Some individuals get little if any nutritive value from their food even if they are eating good raw foods because they have a sluggish or clogged digestive tract. I have microscopically examined blood from people who claim to be eating wholesome foods and found their red blood cells showing signs of malnutrition, lacking in B vitamins, vitamin C, vitamin E and/or iron, calcium and other minerals. This situation arose from long-term neglect of their digestive tracts.

A toxic body combined with the lack of proper nutrition can lead to such illnesses as allergies, chronic fatigue, fibromyalgia, and infertility, among others, in addition to those directly related to the digestive system. Allergies, for example, stem principally from the body's inability to fully and properly digest food. Because of this there are too many strange proteins floating around in the bloodstream, needlessly stimulating the immune system. Then, when another foreign protein such as grass pollen or fruit tree pollen comes along, the body sends histamines to attack it, resulting in an allergic response such as a runny nose or teary eyes. In my experience, the best way to begin fixing allergy problems, is to do a colon and liver cleanse. As much as 90 percent of allergies will clear up with a colon and liver cleanse. The remaining allergies often clear up after adding adrenal support.

The first step to better health, then, is to clean up the digestive tract. After that, or in cases of toxicity elsewhere in the body, there are ways to cleanse other organs, glands and systems. This book is all about cleansing, primarily with essential oils, in order to enjoy the health that is our birthright.

You can't show your best face to the world if your body is constantly struggling with internal health problems, whether or not you are consciously aware of them. That's why the title of this book is "Inner Transformations Using Essential Oils." If you clean up your body on the inside, the changes you create will lead to a whole new outside. You'll feel so much better your whole life will change. Your clean insides will create a clear and vibrant outside!

The following questionnaire presents some symptoms of various organs that might need to be cleaned out or given more nutritional support to help them function better. Mark the questions 1 for mild (occurs infrequently), 2 for moderate (occurs several times a year) or 3 for severe (constant problem). If you have several problem areas, you are a good candidate for cleansing.

1. _____ Butterfly stomach, cramps
2. _____ Eyes or nose watery
3. _____ Eyelids swollen, puffy
4. _____ Indigestion
5. _____ Always hungry
6. _____ Lightheaded often
7. _____ Excessive appetite
8. _____ Hungry between meals
9. _____ Irritable before meals
10. _____ Get "shaky" if hungry
11. _____ Fatigue
12. _____ Urine amount reduced
13. _____ Cold sweats often
14. _____ Sour stomach frequent
15. _____ Acid foods upset
16. _____ Digestion rapid
17. _____ Vomiting frequently
18. _____ Breathing irregular
19. _____ Constipation
20. _____ Diarrhea
21. _____ Constipation alternating with diarrhea
22. _____ Don't perspire
23. _____ Perspire too much
24. _____ Heart palpitates if meal delayed
25. _____ Moody
26. _____ Depression
27. _____ Crave sweets
28. _____ Crave salty foods

29. _____ Sigh frequently
30. _____ Swollen ankles
31. _____ Bruise easily
32. _____ Dizziness
33. _____ Dry skin
34. _____ Burning feet
35. _____ Blurred vision
36. _____ Thinning hair
37. _____ Metallic taste in mouth
38. _____ Nausea
39. _____ Headaches
40. _____ Greasy foods upset
41. _____ Stools light colored
42. _____ Stools greasy
43. _____ Stools extremely loose
44. _____ Stools hard and dry
45. _____ Need to use laxatives
46. _____ Gallstones
47. _____ Bad breath
48. _____ Gas after eating
49. _____ Coated tongue
50. _____ Stomach bloat
51. _____ Insomnia
52. _____ Nervous
53. _____ Can't lose weight
54. _____ Decrease in appetite
55. _____ Dry skin
56. _____ Mental sluggishness
57. _____ Forgetfulness
58. _____ Frequent urination

59. _____ Decreased sex drive			**FEMALES**	
60. _____ Abnormal thirst			1. _____ PMS	
61. _____ Ulcers			2. _____ Painful menses	
62. _____ High blood pressure			3. _____ Painful breasts	

59. _____ Decreased sex drive
60. _____ Abnormal thirst
61. _____ Ulcers
62. _____ High blood pressure
63. _____ Chronic fatigue
64. _____ Suicidal thoughts
65. _____ Tendency to hives
66. _____ Arthritis
67. _____ Brown spots on skin
68. _____ Red moles
69. _____ Allergies
70. _____ Acne
71. _____ Ringing in ears
72. _____ Distended abdomen
73. _____ Frequent colds
74. _____ Drowsy often
75. _____ Weak immune system
76. _____ Varicose veins
77. _____ Itchy skin
78. _____ Excessive falling hair
79. _____ Anemia
80. _____ Joint stiffness after rising

FEMALES
1. _____ PMS
2. _____ Painful menses
3. _____ Painful breasts
4. _____ Menstruate too frequently
5. _____ Periods irregular
6. _____ Vaginal discharge
7. _____ Hot flashes
8. _____ Menses scanty
9. _____ Hair growth on face

MALES
10. _____ Prostate trouble
11. _____ Urination difficult or dribbling
12. _____ Diminished sex drive
13. _____ Anger easily
14. _____ Increased sex drive

To score this questionnaire add up all your points. If you score between 1-10 points your organs probably are functioning pretty well—unless all the symptoms refer to the same organ. If your score is between 10-25 then you would improve your health by beginning with seasonal colon cleansing. If your score is above 25 then it would definitely be to your benefit to begin cleansing now.

REFERENCES

"Poison in Apple Seeds?" Ask a Scientist, Biology Archive, http://www.newton.dep.anl. gov/askasci/bio99/bio99250.htm.

M. Rezaul Haque, J. Howard Bradbury, Total cyanide determination of plants and foods using the picrate and acid hydrolysis methods, Australian National University at Canberra, July 2001. http://www.anu.edu.au/BoZo/CCDN/papers/77_107_114_02.pdf.

William J. Walsh, Ph.D, Biochemical Treatment of Mental Illness and Behavior Disorders, http://www.hriptc.org/BioTreatment.html

The Hidden Dangers of Mega Vitamin C, Alternative Medicine Angel, http://altmedangel. com/arteries.htm

Tim O'Shea, "Ascorbic Acid is not Vitamin C" http://www.newmediaexplorer.org/ sepp/2003/11/17/ascorbic_acid_is_not_vitamin_c.htm.

American Cancer Society: Cancer Facts and Figures 2005. Atlanta, Ga: American Cancer Society, 2005.

Walton Feeds, "Nutritional content of Whole Grains vs. Their Refined Flours" http://www. waltonfeed.com/grain/flour.html

Bernard Jensen, D.C., Tissue Cleansing Through Bowel Management, Escondido, CA 1981

According to Satya Dandekar, PhD, University of California Davis Health System, gut-associated lylmphoid tissue (GALT) accounts for 70 percent of the body's immune system. See http://www.poz.com/articles/761_7786.shtml

"The total mucosal surface area of the adult human GI tract is up to 300 square meters making it the largest body area interacting with the environment....(This) makes the gastrointestinal tract the largest lymphoid or immune organ in the human body. It has been estimated that there are approximately 10 10 (power of 10) immunoglobulin producing cells per meter of small bowel- accounting for approximately 80% of all immunoglobulin producing cells in the body." (Shanahan, F, "The intestinal immune system" in Physiology of the Gastrointestinal Tract, 3rd edition, 1994, ed. Johnson, LR)

Guadalupe, M., et al, Viral Suppression and Immune Restoration in the Gastrointestinal Mucosa of Human Immunodeficiency Virus Type 1-Infected Patients Initiating Therapy during Primary or Chronic Infection, Journal of Virology, Vol. 80, No. 16, Aug. 2006.

Alexander G. Haslberger, "GM Food: The Risk Assessment of Immune Hypersensitivity Reactions Covers More Than Allergenicity", Institute for Microbiology and Genetics, University of Vienna, Austria, Department of food safety, WHO, Geneva, Switzerland. Haslberger states "The role of antigen presenting cells of the gut is now understood to direct immune responses resulting in humoral, cellular or IgE predominant characteristics." See http://www.biotech-info. net/hypersensitivity.html.

CHAPTER 2

To Everything There is a Time and Season

Seasonal Cleansing

According to the Law of the Five Elements, each organ has a time and a season when it receives the most energy from the body. The Law of the Five Elements is a discipline that is thousands of years old, within the fold of traditional Chinese medicine (TCM). It teaches the harmony and inter-relationship of all the organs and energy systems in the body. Energy flows in meridians throughout the entire body, enlivening each organ and meridian in turn. As understood in the Five Elements system, these meridians and their associated organs influence each other in a 24-hour cycle as well as through the cycle of the year; organs are also coupled in yin-yang pairs. Traditional Chinese medicine is a complex approach to understanding the body, but essentially illness is held to be a disruption of the natural energy flow through the meridians. Western medicine is beginning to discover a bio-electric basis for the meridian system, but has not yet accepted the beauty and logic of TCM's holistic approach to health.

When we are cleaning out or strengthening an organ it really helps the body to give the proper supplements to that organ at the proper time. And although you can cleanse the body during any season, especially if you are very sick and need to get well without delay, there are certain seasons when your body will work with you better and help flush out toxins instead of holding on to them.

"The Bodymindspirit tells us to look at Nature as the pattern of the human person so that from Nature we can diagnose and treat. In the season of spring, we do literally sow the seeds for the fall harvest within ourselves. The traditional acupuncturist knows that unless the seeds of healing are sown in their proper season through treatment, the tree—that is the person— will not thrive."

The Law of the Five Elements, Dianne M. Connelly, Ph.D.

Let us look at the earth's seasons and how they affect our bodies and us.

Spring

Spring is really the beginning of the new growing season. The New Year actually used to start around March 25th. It was religious and government politics that changed today's New Year to the middle of winter!

Spring comes and warm weather begins. New plants are springing forth. Most of the edible plants are cleansing plants. Spinaches, violets, and strawberries all have cleansing properties. It is the time of the year for salad greens, which loosen stools. Traditionally, we do our house cleaning in the spring to get rid of the dust, dirt and mud that has collected over winter, and spring is also the time to cleanse our bodies. Our bodies want to shed weight in the spring to get ready for hotter weather and to cool us down. Starting a weight loss or cleansing program in the spring of the year makes sense because our bodies will cooperate with us at that season. The liver and the gall bladder get their major energy allotments in the spring of the year. That is when they want to be cleansed and supported.

Summer

In the summer, the vegetables start growing that build the body. They give us vitamins and minerals necessary to build and heal tissues. So naturally, it is easier for our bodies to heal during the summer. The heart and the small intestine want to be cleansed and supported in the early summer while the spleen (and lymphatics) and the stomach get their energy in the late summer. That is quite logical since these digestive organs need to be able to go to work on the body-building vegetables to extract the vitamins and minerals from them. In addition, by supporting the spleen with proper nutrition during the summer, it will be ready to support the immune system in the fall and winter when the virus season hits.

Fall

Next comes fall. The fall fruits and vegetables are storage foods. They are heavier in their composition. The body uses the squashes and potatoes to put on weight to store fat for the upcoming cold weather. "If there is no autumn harvest, the crops that grow in the summer will rot where they are, without being collected and preserved." <u>The Law of the Five Elements</u>

Speaking of rot, the same thing happens with the food in the colon. If the colon can't handle the foods that it is given in the fall, the foods will rot and putrefy over the winter months, stagnating in the colon. Fall is the time to cleanse and support the colon and the lungs. Supporting the lungs in the fall prepares them for the cold weather ahead when they are under attack from air-borne viruses and the body is perhaps not as vigorous as in warmer months.

Winter

Winter foods are extremely heavy. They are more meaty and fat-laden to keep us warm. Starting a weight loss diet or cleansing program in the winter works against the system and actually makes the body want to put on more weight since it thinks it has been thrown into the starvation mode during the cold months when it already needs to conserve all the energy it can. This is one reason that New Year's weight-loss resolutions often fail: It's simply the wrong time of year.

Our diets are generally more heavily laden with proteins in the winter, so if the kidney isn't cleaned and supported in that season, there is more chance of the body developing gout, which stems from non-digestion of protein products and the deposit of protein wastes into the body tissues instead of elimination through the kidneys.

This doesn't mean that you shouldn't cleanse in the winter, especially if your body is screaming for it! Winter is an excellent time to do a yeast cleanse since the diet required for a yeast cleanse is heavier, consisting of meats and other proteins and little or no starches, sugars or fruits. However, I think that a deep cleanse such as the Master Cleanse would be better advised and more effective in the spring of the year.

The Cleansing Sequence

To get ready for spring cleansing of the body, start in the fall by doing a colon cleanse. Then in the winter clean and support the kidney (and do a yeast cleanse if needed). The colon and kidney need to be ready to take the excess toxins away from the body when the spring comes. Next, start cleaning the liver. If you do not cleanse in this order, when you start the Master Cleanse or a liver cleanse there may be too many toxins for the liver and colon to handle and you will become temporarily sick.

This principle can be illustrated by an actual experience my daughter had in her apartment. One day waste water began backing up in her laundry room, which was on the ground floor. Maintenance workers were unable to fix the problem through their attempts to unclog that drain. Next her kitchen sink began to back up. Then waste water began backing up in another apartment in the complex that was slightly higher in elevation. Nothing the workers tried seemed to work, until they went out into the street and dug up the main sewer. That's where the blockage was. Until they cleared that blockage, no amount of pipe-cleaning would have done any good, and eventually all the apartments on higher floors would also have had backups.

Similarly, a blocked colon, as the main waste pipeline of the body, will not allow toxins to easily exit the body, and no amount of cleansing "upstream" is likely to be really effective until the colon is cleansed. Thus, we cleanse the colon first, followed by the kidney and liver as the other major toxin eliminators, then the various other upstream systems.

By summer you will be ready to eat the body-building vegetables that are ripening then, that will support the body and build the immune system.

Working with the seasons of the year makes perfect sense when cleansing the body. It is a more natural way to live. However, if you have never cleansed your body before and are just now learning how to do it, or if you have been diagnosed with an ailment that cleansing will help, it will not hurt you to cleanse out of season. Still, it is always best to start with a colon cleanse first, then yeast, then kidney, then finish up with the Master Cleanse and a liver cleanse. After the initial cleanout of the body, making seasonal cleansing a pattern to live by for the remainder of your life will keep your body healthy and strong, and you will feel yourself begin to live in harmony with the rhythm of nature.

Time of day

Here is another factor to consider: The 12 main meridians of the body and their associated organs have a beautiful, natural flow of energy that is continuous, around the clock, from one day to the next. When taking supplements for a specific organ it is appropriate to look at the time of day that that organ is most receptive to energy and nourishment.

Admittedly it is difficult to take supplements in the middle of the night. In the case where you need to take a supplement for an organ that gets its energy during the night hours you can take the supplements 12 hours earlier during its complement time. Alternatively, I think it would be better yet to take them 1-3 hours early if that is before your bedtime.

Here is a list of the acupuncture meridians associated with each organ, their times of day and seasons.

Organ	Time	Season
Stomach	7-9 am	late summer
Spleen/Pancreas	9-11 am	late summer
Heart	11 am-1 pm	early summer
Small intestine	1-3 pm	early summer
Bladder	3-5 pm	winter
Kidney	5-7 pm	winter
Circulation/Sex	7-9 pm	early summer
Triple Warmer	9-11 pm	early summer
Gall Bladder	11pm-1 am	spring
Liver	1-3 am	spring
Lung	3-5 am	fall
Large Intestine	5-7 am	fall

There are a few systems that are not mentioned in the meridian seasons, but when studying the laws of TCM it is easy to see where they fit in and where a cleansing regime would be most beneficial. The large intestine meridian fortifies the skin and hair, the kidney fortifies the bones, the stomach and spleen fortify the muscles, the heart meridian fortifies the arteries and the liver fortifies the ligaments. So when supporting these other systems use the times and seasons of their "owner's" meridians.

It is interesting to note that by using the times and seasons chart it is sometimes easier to figure out what is going on with the body. For example, if you wake up every night or fall asleep every afternoon at the same time it may well be a sign that the organ associated with that time is suffering an energy blockage. Of course, there are many things that might be involved, but one good thing you could do is to support that organ with the essential oils and nutrition that it might be lacking.

If you are living a healthy, natural lifestyle, signs and symptoms of an organ dysfunction will usually show up during the time or season that the organ is supposed to be getting its optimum energy. However, it can have a problem at any time and that can show up at any time of the year, especially if your body is already out of kilter. Most people unfortunately are not living as sweet and simple a life as would let them be aware of their meridians anyway. Sometimes when an organ is having problems, the organ that is 12 hours away from it on the clock will be the one evidently acting up! Perhaps it is taking its energy at the wrong time of day. This is called the Midday/Midnight law in Chinese acupuncture. At one time of the day, the organ receives its highest energy. Twelve hours later, it receives its lowest energy. To learn more about seasons and times for organ refer to my book "Ultimate Balance" available through Life Science Publishing.

Other factors

There are many reasons why an organ might not be functioning at its highest level. One important reason, for example, might be that the organ is not getting enough nutrients to support it. I like to refer to what I call the Seven Critical Factors for Radiant Health or if considered in a negative context, the Seven Causes of Disease:

1. The things we eat and drink
2. The air we breathe
3. The way we cleanse
4. The way we rest
5. The way we exercise
6. The thoughts we think
7. The emotions we feel

Eating, drinking or breathing toxins can cripple an organ, or even destroy it. High stress levels tax organs, especially the heart, kidneys and adrenal glands. A misaligned spine might be impairing the nervous system's energy to an under-performing organ. There might exist genetic reasons for the organ's malfunction. The organ may have been damaged physically or chemically. The body's pH might be too low or even too high. Emotions might be playing a part. John Diamond in <u>Life Energy</u> explains that the organs and the emotions work together. It can be difficult to determine whether it was the organ not functioning right that caused the emotional problem, or the emotional problem that caused the organ not to function right. Either way, it is important to fix not only the organ but the associated emotion as well.

In the limbic system of the brain, the neurons for the emotions and the neurons for the organs are next to each other. If a person is in a state of intense emotion, the excess energy produced by this emotion will go into the corresponding organ and be stored there. This energy can change the way the organ functions. Usually this energy is negative energy and wears the organ down. Many times the cause of the disease is the emotion and the disease will not go away until the emotional state that is causing it is corrected.

Some of the emotions associated with the organs are as follows:

Fear, Worry . . . . kidney
Anger, rage . . . . liver, gall bladder
Inner crying . . . . lungs or kidney
Sadness, loss of sweetness. . . . . .pancreas
Lack of joy . . . . heart
Unforgivingness . . . . liver
Revenge . . . . .kidney stones
Stress. stomach (or may affect many systems,
                                                   including the immune system)

To give an example of how the emotions can affect the body, we all know that if we are under stress, we get headaches, our neck and shoulders tighten up and we get mild to severe stomach upset, sometimes to the point of creating ulcers. What is not so easy to see is that hidden, inner crying about some loss can cause the kidney to deposit water into the tissues instead of eliminating it, causing ascites. Ascites can arise from other causes, of course, but prolonged weeping or sadness can often be a factor.

People who do not allow themselves to feel their emotions but bury them or hide them to look stronger to others are at high risk for emotionally- induced disease. A good book to read on this subject is <u>Feelings Buried Alive Never Die</u> by Karol Truman, (available through Life Science Publishing).

On the other hand, if you have a hormonal imbalance, too much estrogen or testosterone can cause high states of unexplained anger, or a lack of progesterone can cause sudden and unexplained crying and depression. It is important when we want to alleviate any disease that we look into all the variables and clean them all up to obtain optimum health.

REFERENCES

Connelly, Dianne M. PhD, Traditional Acupuncture: The Law of Five Elements. Traditional Acupucture Institute Columbia, MD. 1994

Maciocia, Giovanni. The Foundations of Chinese Medicine. Churchill Livingstone Inc. New York, NY 1989

Walther, David S. Applied Kinesiology Synopsis. Systems DC. Pueblo, CO 1988

Kloss, Jethro. Back to Eden. Back To Eden Publishing Co. Loma Linda, CA 1988

Lust, John. The Herb Book. Benedict Lust Publications. 1987

Morter, Dr. Ted Jr. Dynamic Health. Morter Health Systems. Rogers, Ark 1995

Diamond John. Life Energy. Warner Books, Inc NY 1983

Truman, Karol, Feelings Buried Alive Never Die, Olympic Distribution Corp., 1992

Hay, Louise. Heal Your Body. Hay House, Inc. Carlsbad, CA. 1984

CHAPTER 3

Essential Oils: Gold of the Gods

In the previous chapter, we saw how the energy flow to the various organs corresponds to the seasons of the year and times of day. Not only do the organs and meridians of the body correspond to different seasons of the year but also there are certain plants that naturally "belong to" certain organs. Some plants actually resemble different body parts. For example, Hawthorne flowers resemble the heart, a walnut looks like a human brain, a ginseng root may resemble a little man, and a nutmeg looks like an adrenal gland. As is well known in the herbal medicine world, ginseng is a general body tonic, the Hawthorne berry supports the heart; walnuts contain fatty acids that support the brain, and nutmeg oil has been shown to have corticosteroid activity that would support the adrenals.

Although the correspondence between a plant and an organ or function is not usually this obvious, herbalists have always searched out and noted which herbs help which systems of the body.

For thousands of years, different cultures around the globe have been using herbs and essential oils to heal and cleanse the body. However, it has only been very recently that essential oils have been brought to the attention of Western society. In ancient Egypt, essential oils were considered the "gold of the gods." Only kings and queens could afford the luxury of using essential oils. Servants would take the leaves or other plant parts that were being distilled for oils and infuse them into teas or extract them in alcohol for their own personal use.

In the past, our culture and other cultures, like the American Indian or the Chinese, knew what plants would help a person and what plants could poison a person. However, modern Western culture, on the other hand, has preferred to experiment with unnatural synthetic chemicals for health care.

One of the problems with synthetic drugs is that they are unnatural; the body was not designed with them in mind and doesn't know how to metabolize them, so they get stuck in the body (see the section on skin in Chapter 9). Another is that they always have so many "effects." The one the doctors want is called the "therapeutic effect" and the other, unwanted ones are called "side effects," but they all come with the drug. The side effects sometimes cause so much trouble the patient has to take another drug just to deal with them—and perhaps yet another drug to deal with the side effects of that one.

Another problem with drugs is that the body adapts to them as best it can, and so do bacteria, so that the drugs lose their effectiveness over time. Drugs also tend to merely suppress the symptoms, or force the disease inward where it continues to live sub-clinically, whereas natural remedies help body systems overpower and eliminate the source of the disease.

Within the last few years, more and more research has been done on the health benefits of essential oils. These oils are where the healing power of the plant resides. Dr. John Christopher, a leading herbalist in the United States in the 20th century, used to travel around the U.S. teaching about the healing power of plants. According to Dr. Christopher, the body assimilates the herb best in tea, extract or tincture form better than in pill form. The reason for this, he explained, is that the essential oil is released from the plant during hot water infusion or while soaking in alcohol and it is the essential oil that holds the constituents that support and heal the body.

Actually, essential oils have been found to be far more powerful and effective than dried or fresh herbs. The reason is that there is only a minute amount of oil in each plant. Remember, that is where the healing power resides. Therefore, when a cup of tea or a capsule of herb is taken, only a small quantity of the healing constituents is made available to the body. On the other hand, when a large quantity of plants is processed to distill their essential oils, the result is a much more potent product than even a mound of raw herb would be—assuming that all that herb could ever be swallowed.

It takes a pound of peppermint leaves to yield just a few drops of Peppermint oil. Moreover, peppermint has one of the highest yields of all the herbs. Some essential oils, like Rose oil, require enormous quantities of plant material to yield just a few ounces of oil.

A spokeswoman at Young Living Farms told me that one acre of peppermint yields approximately 3 tons of peppermint herb which in turn yields between 80 -120 lbs. of Peppermint oil. But consider this about the herb Melissa: "it can take 2-3 tons of Melissa plant material to produce one pound of Melissa oil... It takes 5,000 pounds of rose petals to produce approximately one pint (less than a pound) of rose oil," according to the Essential Oils Desk Reference. As you can see, essential oils are very potent and just one drop of oil will do more for you than would several cups of tea, and far more than would a handful of capsules of dried herb.

How to use essential oils

There are many different methods of using essential oils. Here are some of the most common and effective I use for my patients and myself.

◆ To make a big change quickly (for low adrenal function, stomach flu or sinus problems), I do what I call the **Jump Start**, as follows: Take one drop of essential oil by mouth every minute for 10 minutes, then one drop by mouth every 10 minutes for an hour, then one drop by mouth every waking hour for the rest of the day. If you rub the drop in the buccal mucosa (inner cheek lining) of the mouth, it doesn't leave such a bitter or tangy taste as it would on the tongue, and it is also absorbed more readily. You can always use a chaser like a piece of bread or a glass of water to rid yourself of the oil taste if you don't like it.

◆ CAUTION: If you are going to use essential oils orally you should do so under the care of a trained health professional. Not all essential oils can be used orally. And most essential oils are not pure enough to be used internally. It is extremely important that you use only therapeutic-grade oils that have been organically grown and steam-distilled. This will insure that you don't ingest chemical fertilizers, herbicides, pesticides used in growing the plants or chemical solvents or other toxins used in processing the oils.

◆ Another milder method for beginning to use essential oils is the Vita Flex method with foot reflexology points (see Appendix A): Put the oils on the points and then roll the fingers across those points, from pad of finger-to-finger nail. This method is taught in the Essential Oils Desk Reference. When I first started with the oils I only put them on the foot reflexology points and the organ alarm points. (These are essentially just over the organ on the body. See Appendix A.) I did get results but it would take several months to see them. I found that taking oils by mouth in the lining of the cheek was a quicker way to achieve the results I wanted. In addition if you combine these two methods you get even quicker results! (refer to my book, "Ultimate Balance".

◆ In addition to reflexology points, you can apply the oils on the skin at the afflicted site, diluted, if the oils are strong ones or undiluted if they are mild ones. A helpful dilution chart is also found in the Essential Oils Desk Reference. Always test the oils on your skin. If a particular oil gives any burning sensations, dilute it with V-6, almond, olive or even vegetable oil.

◆ Never put oils in the eyes. **If an oil accidentally gets in the eye, put olive or almond oil (even cooking oil in an emergency) in the eye to dilute it, and then wipe it out. Never try to wash oils out with water—it will only make it worse.**

◆ My favorite way is the French method taught by Dr. Penëol. He recommends taking 1-2 drops of oil frequently throughout the day. I find it quite effective to simultaneously apply a drop of oil on the foot reflexology points or on the alarm point of the organ that you want to affect, and then take one drop by mouth (rubbing it on the inside of the cheek). Repeat 3 or 4 times a day.

◆ You can put essential oils in bath water to soak in them. Most people who are not used to the strength of the oils mix them with a 1-2 tbsp. of bath gel or Epsom salts before putting them in the water because some of these oils can sting if they come in contact with delicate membrane areas.

◆ I love to soak in Clove oil or Aroma Seiz for tight muscles or Peace and Calming to calm my nerves. You can also soak in a few drops of Peppermint to reduce fevers or Thieves oil to help combat flu's or colds. (These are all from Young Living Essential Oils.)

◆ If I want to make an emotional change or quickly help the brain, I find that smelling the oils is the perfect way, either directly out of the open bottle or by rubbing a drop under my nose that I then can smell with every breath. Aromas go immediately and directly to the brain. (See Appendix A)

◆ Though this should always be done under the care of a trained health professional, it is possible to take essential oils—diluted 50% with a quality vegetable oil—in capsules to treat an organ system or disease state. I prefer to administer the oils in a single drop via the inner lining of the cheek as it doesn't take as much oil, doesn't tend to come back up in burps, and gets into the blood faster. However, whenever aches and fevers start, I often prescribe taking diluted Oregano oil for one or two nights in a row to help get over the illness faster.

Don't forget that for some purposes you can also put capsules in the rectum or vagina. If used in the vagina it is important to dilute the oils even further as they will burn. I usually use a dilution of 7 drops essential oil per tablespoon of olive oil.

◆ You can make warm or cold compresses with the oils. When cleansing the kidneys, for example, it is very soothing to put Rosemary, Sage and Juniper oils directly over the kidneys (on the back) and then put a warm wet towel on top of that for about 15 minutes.

◆ I use a cold compress when there has been ligament or muscle tearing or stretching. Put the chosen oils on the painful area and an ice pack on top. I suggest Idaho Balsam Fir, Lemongrass, Cypress or Lavender.

When cleansing, you can choose any of these methods of using essential oils. If there is a specific oil that I think is best for dealing with a particular organ or cleanse, I will point it out in the text.

As mentioned in the introduction, I prefer Young Living Essential Oils. I have had excellent results both on myself and in treating my patients using these oils. We have experimented with other brands and have not had the same results. For example, I have treated many Amish patients who do not vaccinate their children. They tend to get a lot of childhood diseases in their communities. There was a pertussis outbreak in several communities a few years ago. I told several families in different communities to take one drop of Oregano and mix it with a teaspoon of butter and put it on toast to give to the child to eat three times a day. Usually the child can sleep better the first night because the coughing has decreased. By the third day the children are usually well. In one community, this didn't seem to be working. One of the fathers called me and said that the oregano oil didn't work. I asked him what brand he was using. He said that it was an inexpensive brand that he found at a health food store. He thought he would use it instead of the more expensive Young Living brand. I told him that that was why it wasn't working. It was probably diluted or not pure or not distilled properly so that it didn't have the right constituents to heal the body.

It is imperative that you use a therapeutic-grade essential oil that is steam-distilled under low pressure. Not only will this type of oil retain all the original, natural constituents but it will also be free from chemical solvents that might otherwise have been used to harvest the oil from the plant. Since many of the solvents used to process lesser-quality oils are oil-soluble there is a good chance that they will stay in the oil and be conveyed to your body and tissues when you ingest the oil or put it on your skin. (To learn more about therapeutic grade oils and how oils are distilled and processed from the plant see the Essential Oils Desk Reference compiled by Essential Science Publishing.)

Throughout this book, I will be referencing the single essential oils, essential oil blends and nutritional products produced by Young Living Essential Oils. Young Living's oils have an energy or electricity that I have not seen nor felt in other oils. I have looked at several different brands of essential oils under a dark-field microscope. Essential oils from Young Living have a sparkle and "light show" effect that is like watching a distant fireworks display or sometimes gazing at the night sky. They move and sparkle. This tells me that they are alive. Other oils seem dead in that you cannot tell any difference between them and plain old cooking oil under the microscope. There is no sparkle, no lightshow, nothing but a blank field. If you are certain that a particular oil from a different company is a high quality essential oil, feel free to use it. But you may not get the same results. If after 2 months you have not achieved good results using the brand of oils that you have chosen, then I highly recommend that you switch to Young Living Essential Oils. Be forewarned, you usually get what you pay for. A lot goes into a top-quality essential oil, and it's worth what it costs.

Appendix B at the back of the book contains a chart showing which Young Living essential oils and supplements support each organ we will be discussing in this book.

REFEENCES

Rodale's Encyclopedia of Herbs, Kowalchik & Hylton, Ed. Rodale Press, Emmaus, PA 1987

Kloss, Jethro, Back to Eden, Back to Eden Publishing Co., Loma Linda, CA 1988

Lust, John, The Herb Book, Bantom Books, New York NY, 1987

Essential Desk Reference, Essential Science Publishing

Rishel, Jonas,The Indian Physician (reprint), Ohio State University, 1980.

* All products mentioned in this and the following paragraphs are from Young Living Essential Oils unless otherwise noted.

CHAPTER 4

The Colon: Don't Block the Exit
(FALL)

One of the most well-known sayings in the world of alternative health care is "Death begins in the colon." This saying is frequently quite true. Hippocrates himself said "All disease begins in the gut." Let's take a quick look at the digestive system, working our way down to the colon, and see why that would be so.

How Digestion Works

The digestive tract starts in the mouth and actually is just one long tube from mouth to anus. It changes size, shape and function along the way. It has valves that close to keep the food in one area or another for a while to go through certain functions before another valve opens to let it pass to go to the next part of the tract, and smooth muscle tissue to move it along. Nevertheless, it is essentially just one long tube, and it is the primary way that things get into our bodies, whether food or non-food.

The mouth's main job is to masticate the food into small enough particles that the rest of the digestive tract will be able to break it down into nutrients. No other part of the digestive tract has teeth, therefore it is important to chew the food well so that it can mix with the enzymes that will be released later on in the digestive process. Many times the cause of indigestion is simply failure to chew food sufficiently so that the rest of the digestive tract can perform its functions properly. For example, the cells in fruits and vegetables have indigestible cellulose walls that must be broken down by the action of the teeth so the small intestine can mix enzymes with those plant foods to digest them.

Another of the mouth's functions is to mix saliva with the food. An amylase enzyme called ptyalin is released into the saliva by the parotid glands to begin breaking down simple sugars and starches, and there are also enzymes to begin fat digestion and to attack bacteria. The saliva then eases the food's passage down the esophagus.

Additionally, the process of chewing signals the other digestive organs, via the nervous system, to get ready to do their jobs. So, all in all, Mom's advice to chew your food thoroughly was exactly right.

From the mouth the bolus of masticated food moves down the esophagus into the stomach. The cardiac or esophageal valve at the upper end of the stomach and the pyloric valve at the bottom end of the stomach close so the stomach can mix the swallowed matter with hydrochloric acid and pepsin. Their purpose is to begin the process of breaking down proteins in the food. Proteins have a complex structure and it takes several steps to compete their digestion. (Later, enzymes will be added by the pancreas and small intestine to further break down the proteins.) Meanwhile, the enzymes added by the saliva continue to work on carbohydrate digestion until overcome by the stomach's acidity.

At the end of this process, which takes several hours, the pyloric valve opens, gradually releasing the partially-digested food, now called chyme, into the small intestine. There it is mixed with a bicarbonate solution and enzymes to neutralize the acidity created in the stomach and to continue the breakdown of proteins, fats and sugars. Further along in the small intestine, absorption of nutrients begins to take place.

The chyme passes through the small intestine in segments. It is churned and propelled along by smooth-muscle contractions. The chyme stays in the first section of the small intestine, called the duodenum, for several hours being churned and mixed with enzymes until the nutrients are ready to be absorbed. These enzymes are produced by the pancreas, liver and the small intestine itself, to break down the complex molecules of fats, proteins and carbohydrates into simple molecules that the cells of the body can use. The chyme subsequently passes into the second section of the small intestine, called the jejunum, where most nutrient absorption takes place. If the food was not sufficiently chewed in the mouth, it may pass through the stomach, small intestine and colon only partially digested since it wasn't able to mix thoroughly with the enzymes and break down into nutrients.

The third and last section of the small intestine, the ileum, primarily houses immune system cells, along with a small amount of bacteria, that protect us from pathogenic microorganisms we have ingested. When we acknowledge that 80 percent of the immune system is in the digestive tract, this is the location of a good part of it, so Hippocrates' statement is true not only of the colon, but the stomach and small intestine too.

Next the ileocecal valve opens and the chyme passes into the first section of the large intestine (colon), called the cecum. It's called the ileocecal valve because it controls the passage from the ileum to the cecum, and it can be a locus of problems, on occasion. At times it may be "stuck" open or closed and need adjustment by a chiropractor or other healthcare practitioner. Another troublesome bit of gut anatomy, the appendix, also resides in this neighborhood. Some say the appendix is unnecessary, because they can't figure out what purpose it has, but recently it has been proposed that the appendix may be the repository of beneficial colon bacteria, from which the colon can be replenished with this "good" bacteria following a bout of diarrhea or other illness. We will discuss these colonic bacteria a little later.

After entering the colon, the chyme is moved along in a process called peristalsis and is squeezed to extract its water and electrolytes. The body efficiently recycles most of the water and electrolytes that reach the colon, as well as the bile salts. The large intestine is rich with blood vessels to carry nutrients, locally-produced vitamins and water away.

Causes of Constipation

A major cause of constipation is not drinking enough water so that as the body extracts the water it requires from the chyme, you end up with very hard and dry stools. The importance of fiber can be seen in this connection too: Fiber retains water, keeping the stool soft and easy to pass. Consuming plenty of fiber and plenty of water is one of the true keys to good health. How much? C. Everett Koop, former Surgeon General of the United States, recommended 35 grams of fiber, while other sources recommend 20-30 grams. The average American gets less than 20 grams per day, not nearly enough. For colon function, we are talking about insoluble fiber, the kind found in whole grains, vegetables and various other things like strawberry seeds and popcorn hulls. As we will see in discussing the microorganisms of the colon in Chapter 5, soluble fiber is vital for our health too, but, unlike the insoluble kind, it doesn't add bulk to the stool, which is our focus here.

The standard for water intake per day is eight 8-oz. glasses, or some say a quart per 50 pounds of body weight. Anyone who is not aware of how much fiber and how much water they presently consume is most likely not getting enough. For starters, simply eat more fiber and drink more water. An excellent suggestion is to begin taking one tsp of ICP twice a day. Having said that, let me also state that it is possible in extreme cases to go overboard and get too much fiber and too much water, tying up nutrients so they can't be absorbed, or even leaching them out of the body. But the vast majority of people are in no danger of overdoing it.

The large intestine is filled with mucous glands, the purpose of which is to coat the chyme so it can pass over the villi of the large intestine easier, and also to protect itself from drugs, heavy metals and other harmful matter. (The villi, tiny finger-like projections on the inside of the colon, are where the absorption of nutrients takes place.) Certain unnatural, processed foods, like pasteurized milk products, cause these glands to over-produce mucus. Other artificial foods like white flour products, when mixed with this mucus, create a gluey substance that coats the walls of the colon. This coating is then baked on in the 100° oven of the colon. If you have ever made Christmas ornaments or other crafts with your children by mixing white flour and milk, then slow-baking the resulting clay, you know just how hard this substance can become! Not only is it hard like cement but it is virtually immovable so that the peristalsis of the colon slows down and practically stops, not allowing the contents to move forward and leave the colon through the anus. This prevention of normal peristalsis is another cause of constipation.

The Problems of a Toxic Colon

In extreme cases, the colon can become so clogged as a result of poor dietary choices and insufficient fiber and water intake that the colon expands with the mucoid plaque and excess fecal matter to become a megacolon as much as 5 times the colon's normal size, and weighing up to 40 lbs, even though the passageway through may be only pencil-thin. And the weight of an overloaded transverse colon (the part that crosses over from the right to the left side of the body) can cause it to prolapse and press down on the uterus and ovaries in women, or on the prostrate gland in men, leading to infection, infertility and other reproductive problems. It can also press on the bladder, causing discomfort and infection. Prolapse can also lead to dangerous adhesions between the various organs.

Even worse, toxins that are retained too long in a clogged colon can fester and create a wide range of disease processes, including cancer. Dr. Anthony Badzier, a professor of gastroenterology in New York, states, "After concluding a 25 year study of over 5,000 cases, every physician should realize that intestinal toxins are the most important primary and contributing causes of many disorders and health problems of the human body." Dr William Hunter states, "The colon is the sewer system of the body, but with neglect and abuse, it becomes a cesspool of toxins that spill over into the body." The Royal Medical Society of Great Britain concluded that more than 65 different health problems are caused by a toxic colon. This is probably a conservative estimate. Scientific studies have shown diseases as diverse as arthritis, fibromyalgia, dermatitis, fatigue and even many mental problems to improve with care of the lower colon, aside from more predictable ailments of the colon itself.

The Problem of Parasites
Another serious ailment that occurs when this thick lining is blocking the absorption of nutrients and the contents are not moving along rapidly is a parasitic infestation. The parasites live on the stuff you eat and are unable to digest or pass (especially sugars and starches), and in return excrete toxins that make you sick. Hardly seems like a fair deal, does it? Yet the typical American may unwittingly have all kinds of vermin living in his or her intestine, happily eating and breeding and creating disease. In fact, by some estimates, humans may host as many as 100 different parasites, including hookworms, tapeworms, roundworms, pinworms, flukes, amoebas and giardia and other types of protozoa. They may live in the bowel or throughout the body, usually migrating back and forth to the colon. They can lay eggs by the scores of thousands every day. They cause a multitude of diseases (some of which are listed later in this chapter), and rob you of vitality. Some types of parasites may also perforate the bowel, allowing bits of proteins, for example, to escape undigested into the abdomen. This then leads to various allergies, because allergies are a sensitivity to foreign proteins. And it isn't just undigested food particles that leak through the intestinal wall, but non-food particles that may have been ingested as well as bits of fecal matter. This is a way that all manner of micro-organisms and foreign matter can potentially find access to the blood and to body tissues, creating toxicity.

But when I see a person who has intestinal parasites and who also needs a colon cleanse, I will usually have them clean up the colon first before attacking the parasite problem. The reason for this is that if the colon is still clogged when the parasites are flushed out, they will just return to feast on the leftover muck! They can do that because there are still hiding places for them and their eggs and cysts in the colon, and they also migrate to and from other organs of the body. Even if by diligent effort they were all killed, conditions are still ideal for them to re-establish themselves if (or really, *when*) reacquired from either within or outside of the body. Therefore, I will return to the subject of eliminating parasites later in the chapter, after discussing the mechanics of colon cleansing.

Another reason "death begins in the colon" is because a toxic colon pushes toxins to the other organs of elimination, such as the liver and kidneys, creating disease processes there. If not eliminated, they can wind up being stored as miniature vectors of toxicity. Eventually even the skin becomes recruited as the last-ditch organ of elimination, leading to blemishes and skin diseases as toxins are pushed out of the body. Brain function is impaired as well by blood-borne toxins. All these problems begin in the colon. An unhealthy colon drags the entire body down with it.

Clean it up!

In doing a cleanse you need to take the right type of herbs and oils that will push the intestinal contents along, restoring the normal motility of the colon, and you also need enzymes that will break up the mucus and the lining of the bowel. Many people just take laxatives that will relax the colon or thin the fecal matter so that it is easier to move. The problem with a laxative is that it disturbs the muscle tone of the colon and causes it to decrease its activity. The body eventually becomes dependent on laxatives.

Other people become dependent on enemas. If they continue to take enemas to get the stool out, once again the action of the muscles is toned down since they don't have to work as much and the colon becomes lazy. I recommend enemas as a way to deliver nutrients to the body quickly, but not as the answer to the problem of a gunked-up colon, because the water tends just to flush out what is loose in the bowel without affecting what is clinging to the sides.

Sometimes a person's colon is so blocked up the only solution seems to be to get a hydrocolonic treatment. This involves injecting a large quantity of water at high pressure via the rectum that can move all through the colon and help clean out blockages. But even if one in desperation resorts to a hydrocolonic treatment, it is still necessary to do a colon cleanse to break up the hard material clinging to the walls of the colon and restore it to its natural, healthy condition. That stuff is still there, even after a hydrocolonic wash-out.

To understand how to cleanse, you need to know what your goal is. You probably eat 3 meals a day, so shouldn't you have 3 bowel movements? Where do you think that stuff is if you don't get rid of it all day, or for several days, or a week or more? Well, as a matter of fact, most people carry around at least 7 pounds of stagnant, impacted fecal matter in their colons. Yuck! The goal for good colon function is 2 to 3 bowel movements a day that are fast and easy to pass, well formed and float in the toilet. So you cleanse to achieve that goal. Some people take 6 weeks to get there; others take up to a year. The majority of people take about 3 months. But it's not quite as simple as having several bowel movements a day. According to Dr. Bernard Jensen, a leader in the field of herbal cleansing for 50 years, you should cleanse until you pass what he describes as the lining coating the bowel, or, in other words, the mucoid plaque. It is black and long and holds together in a long tube shape, and it consists of all the caked material that had been lining the bowel and making it difficult for the bowel to function as it was designed to. Once that passes, the bowel automatically begins to function properly. Once that passes you have achieved your goal.

A good colon cleanse is well balanced to support the kidneys and liver while you are cleansing. A lot of toxins are released while cleansing that upon entering the blood stream or liver make you nauseous, headachy, weak or sick. A well balanced colon cleanse will have herbs in it that break up mucus, release the caked-on lining from the bowel, absorb toxins so they don't get into the bloodstream, stimulate peristaltic action and add bulk to help move the intestinal contents through the system. Some of the herbs and oils typically found in a good cleanse are: German chamomile flowers, cascara sagrada, bentonite, diatomaceous earth, psyllium seed, fennel seed, burdock root, garlic, barberry root bark, (echinacea purpurea) root, ginger root, apple pectin, licorice root, cayenne pepper, the essential oils of rosemary (Rosmarinus officinalis CT 1,8 cineol), tarragon (Artemisia dracunculus), peppermint (Mentha piperita), ginger (Zingiber officinale), anise (Pimpinella anisum. Psyllium seed powder, oat bran, flax seed, and fennel seed.

The cleanse that I recommend is from Young Living Essential Oils. It's called Cleansing Trio and it is simply a kit of Comfortone, ICP and Essentialzyme all in one, for slightly less than buying these three products separately. In addition to being effective as a cleanse it has enzymes to help you digest your food until the body can do it on its own. Another reason I recommend Young Living's colon cleanse is that it tastes good and doesn't make you sick while you take it. That can be a pretty important factor in your successful completion of a cleanse! Some other colon cleanses are not well balanced with the ingredients necessary to support the liver and kidney and, as a result, a person might become quite nauseous, achy, headachy or gassy. You want the toxins to leave your body, not be put back into the circulation.

While on Young Living's cleanse you regulate it according to your own body's needs. Everyone is different as to how much of the colon cleanse they need, so you get to make your own adjustments. You really have to experiment with it. If you have any concerns, by all means do your cleanse under the supervision of a good natural healthcare practitioner.

There are a few different ideas on the mechanics of how to colon cleanse. Some are gentler than others. For example, one healer suggests that you take eight to ten capsules of the cleanser the first day to "blast it out," if you will. From there you decrease the amount that you are taking by a pill a day. I personally think that that would be a good approach for someone who is having great difficulty with constipation and can afford to be at home near the toilet all day for several days. It does clean the colon faster then the more gentle method below, but it is possible that the person could become quite sick to the stomach and also have a severe headache from the sudden release of toxins evoked by this method. I recommend that if the more gentle method described below does not work for you, try the above method to see what it can accomplish. **With either method, you should drink three quarts (12 8-oz. glasses) of water a day.** It sounds like a lot, but it is quite doable. One easy method is to simply have enough portable water bottles at hand to add up to 3 quarts (or 3 liters, which is a little more, but is probably the way you will find most bottled water measured nowdays), and drink them throughout the day. This will also greatly benefit your kidneys. If you just absolutely can't drink that much, at least drink two quarts. You need to drink water religiously while on the cleanse, or else all the fiber you'll be taking will create a blockage rather than an easy bowel movement.

The way I usually suggest that my patients colon cleanse is to start with one Comfortone* capsule in the morning. The next day take a capsule in the morning and another at night. Increase by one capsule a day alternating day and night until you are getting two or three bowel movements a day. The Comfortone is designed to restore peristalsis to the colon. Don't be alarmed if your intestines get "gurgley" and perhaps even slightly sore as the Comfortone creates activity where there once was only stagnation.

If you have been doing all this for a week and still haven't achieved two or three BM's a day, add a drop or two of Peppermint oil to a glass of your water or Vitaflex it into your feet and see if that helps. Taking about 1/2 to 2 tsp of Natural Calm a day will also assist the bowels in moving. Try a little before you try a lot, because it can be quite a laxative! Further, I have seen people not getting enough essential fatty acids into the gut so it is "dehydrated". Fatty meats and fish help there, or you can go the supplement route. Butter plays an important role in the gut flora, so eat all you can. Life-5 from YLO also helps. Sometimes the problem is that the low back and pelvic bones need to be adjusted by a Chiropractor to get the proper nerve function working to the area.

After you have achieved the healthy state of two or three good bowel movements a day, begin taking 1 tsp of ICP in the mornings in addition to the Comfortone. ICP is a proprietary blend of fiber and herbs created to provide bulk and nutrition. The best way to use it is to stir it into juice or water and drink it down quickly, before it gets thick. Add ½ tsp of ICP a day until you are achieving large bulky stools but are not constipated. Gary Young suggests that you continue adding ICP until you get to 1 Tbs a day in the morning and 1 Tbs a day at night. The Comfortone activates your bowel, while the ICP adds bulk and some scouring action to carry the gunk away. Again, you really need to drink your water faithfully to keep this stuff moving along. Taking one Essentialzyme (NOT Essentialzymes-4, that's a different product) between meals also helps break up the plaque in the colon and absorb toxins. Essentialzyme is packed full of enzymes for that purpose. Continue on with the ICP, Comfortone and Essentialzyme until you have completely cleansed your colon, passed the "lining" described above and are having two or three good, easy bowel movements a day. To reiterate, this will likely take months, so stay with it, it's worth it.

Step-by-step

Here is a step-by-step outline of the gentle method described above:

1. Begin with 1 ComforTone in the morning. The second day take one in the morning and one in the evening. The third day take two in the morning and one in the evening, then two in the morning and two in the evening and so on, building up to a maximum of 10 daily. Remember that your goal is 2 to 3 bowel movements a day that are fast and easy to pass, well formed and float in the toilet. When you reach that goal you don't need to add any more capsules daily. Stay on that level until you pass the mucoid plaque. If you are having diarrhea, decrease your capsules until your bowels are firm again. If you are having constipation, decrease your capsules until your bowels are easier to pass or add magnesium, peppermint oils or get an adjustment from a chiropractor.

    Along with the ComforTone, take Essentialzyme caplet 3 times daily, between meals. Drink your water!

2. When having 2-3 good bowel movements daily begin taking ICP, 1 tsp in the morning. Mix it with juice and drink it down quickly. Add ½ tsp per day until you reach 1 Tbsp. (3 tsp.) in the morning and 1 Tbsp. in the evening. Stay on ComforTone and Essentialzyme. Keep drinking lots of water!

3. Continue colon cleansing until the mucoid plaque drops out of the colon. This may take between 6 weeks and 18 months. To help speed the cleansing along, it is a good idea to use the Large Intestine energy balance from "Ultimate Balance".

 Scan the QR Code to find out more about the mucoid plaque.

While on the colon cleanse you can take whatever supplements you want to take. Many people want to know what they should eat while on a colon cleanse. I generally don't put people on a different diet while cleansing but it doesn't hurt to change to a more natural and healthy diet. The cleanse will begin to assist you in changing your diet naturally as your body will be drawn to healthier food. I will also point you toward healthy choices throughout the book.

The cleanse takes care of the problem for good if you change your diet and eat less white flour products and more fruits and vegetables and whole-wheat/whole-grain products. If you don't change your diet, milk and white flour will again create a paste in the colon that coats the inside and makes it unable to function properly. This is the leading cause of colon cancer. After cleaning up your colon do you want to risk that again? Some people do choose to continue to eat white flour products (it seems to be in most manufactured foods, not just bread) and drink milk and then cleanse every 6 months to deal with the problem, but I personally feel that the wiser choice is to drink water or fruit juice and eat whole-grain foods that have more nutrients and are healthier for the body.

Cleaning Up the Parasites

After you have achieved a clean, functioning colon, it's time to get rid of the parasites that have been living there. Of course parasites are not restricted to the colon; they typically are found throughout the body, but the main entry is through the digestive tract, and a stagnant colon is their home base and prime breeding ground. Or <u>was</u>, now that you've cleaned it up!

Symptoms of a parasitic infestation can include such diverse ailments as:

- AIDS
- Allergies
- Anal Itching
- Anemia
- Arthritis
- Bloating
- Blood sugar imbalances
- Bruxism (grinding teeth)
- Chronic fatigue
- Confusion
- Constipation
- Degenerative muscle diseases
- Depression
- Diarrhea
- Eczema
- Endometriosis
- Gas (upper and lower)
- Gluten intolerance
- Hypoglycemia
- Hypothyroidism
- Immune system impairment
- Irritable bowel syndrome
- Itchy skin or nose
- Joint pain
- Memory loss
- Nervousness
- Rashes
- Sleep disorders
- Sugar cravings
- Vitamin B-12 and folic acid deficiency

I recommend Para Free from Young Living Essential Oils because it is the best remedy I have ever used, and it is effective against parasites wherever they may be in the body. I did an experiment once with some of my patients who had blood flukes. We could see the little worms swimming in their blood through the dark-field microscope. I put three of them on Para Free gel caps as directed on the bottle. I put five of them on a tincture of wormwood, black walnut, pumpkin seeds and cayenne pepper, which is an accepted herbal remedy for parasites. We drew blood (finger sticks) every day to see what happened. In three days, the flukes had disappeared from the blood of the people who were taking the Para Free. It took two weeks for the flukes to disappear from the blood of the patients taking the tincture. I had both groups continue on their regime for a total of 9 weeks to make sure that all the eggs, cysts, and larvae were killed. I checked their blood at 12 weeks and the parasites were still gone in both groups. Both remedies worked, but the Para Free worked much more quickly and was definitely easier to swallow.

One of my patients had amoebas, and had had constant diarrhea for 3 years. She had been on every drug that her medical doctor could think of to try to get rid of the amoebas. Nothing helped. She then decided to try herbs. She was on anti-parasitic herbs for a year without success before she came to me. I told her about Para Free and she bought some and used it. Within 3 weeks her diarrhea was gone and she felt much better. I told her to finish the bottle. After she did, she went to her doctor who ran all the tests and declared that she was free from amoebas.

The instructions on the Para Free bottle suggest that you take 4 gel caps two times a day. You are to do this for 3 weeks, rest a week and then repeat the 3 weeks, rest another week and then repeat the course one last time. Many people complain that they burp up oils all day while taking Para Free. If this is a problem for you, take 2 gel caps four times a day along with some food. Many times this helps keep you from burping the oils. Originally Para Free was available only as a liquid intended for rectal use, about an ounce of the liquid to be squirted into the rectum at night. Doing it that way is much cheaper and you don't burp oils at all. Gary Young made the formula into gel caps because so many people complained about having to put the oils in the rectum. But this would seem to be the better approach, since that is the closest point to where the majority of parasites are. I have inserted the gel caps into babies' rectums as a suppository and it was very effective against parasites. I suggest it would work equally well for adults as a faster way to deliver the Para Free than the oral route, and easier to do than a liquid enema.

Another thing to consider is that parasites' life cycle includes reproducing in the colon at the time of the full moon. Of course they can't see the full moon, but they must feel it, because they head for the colon at that time to lay their eggs. Herbalists suggest using their parasite protocols to coincide with the time of the full moon, for at least one or two moon cycles, for that reason. Para Free, on the other hand, will eliminate parasites any time, anywhere in the body, which is another great reason to use it rather than an herbal blend.

Many times people see parasites in the toilet while taking Para Free. Others may never see anything, but stool samples show that the parasites are gone.

In some areas it is wise to deworm every 6 months. Some parts of the country are more prone to parasite infestation. I would certainly take Para Free with me if traveling in another country. People who own pets should also plan on taking Para Free frequently, as it is quite easy to pick up parasites or their eggs unsuspectingly from an animal. Anyone who has pets, works with animals or goes camping or swimming in the wild would likewise be well-advised to do a parasite cleanse often. I had a client who lived with cats and also enjoyed camping and kayaking over the course of many years. She was not aware of the danger of parasitic infestation, and eventually discovered worms of different kinds all over her body. At that point she was more than eager to do a parasite cleanse!

Another important factor in preventing an infestation or re-infestation is to strictly avoid eating undercooked meats and fish and unwashed vegetables. We've all seen news accounts of people who have gotten sick from eating something as healthy as salad. Sadly, organically raised vegetables may be even more likely to harbor parasites, since they may have been grown with "natural fertilizer" (read, manure) and haven't been treated with chemicals of any kind.) You would also be wise to purify your drinking water, not only to get rid of parasites but to filter out chemicals. Finally, it wouldn't hurt to follow up every colon cleanse with a parasite cleanse.

Now, congratulations on having a clean, well-functioning colon, the first step to better health!

---

* All products mentioned in this and the following paragraphs are from Young Living Essential Oils.

REFERENCES

Guyton, Arthur C. Textbook of Medical Physiology. W.B. Saunders Co., Philadelphia PA 1991

Walther D.C., David S., Applied Kinesiology Synopsis, Systems DC, Pueblo CO 1988

Koop M.D., C. Everett, The Surgeon General's Report on Nutrition and Health: Summary and Recommendations, Diane Books Publishing Company 1988

Christopher, John H., Dr. Christopher Talks On Rejuvenation Through Elimination, self-published Springville UT 1976

Jensen D.C., Bernard, Dr. Jensen's Guide to Better Bowel Care, Avery Publishing Group, Rev. Ed. 1988.

Essential Desk Reference, Essential Science Publishing

Jensen D.C., Bernard, Tissue Cleansing Through Bowel Management, Bernard Jensen 1981

Anti M, et al. Water supplementation enhances the effect of high-fiber diet on stool frequency and laxative consumption in adult patients with functional constipation. Hepatogastroenterology. 1998 May-Jun;45(21):727-32.

Pereira MA, et al. Dietary fiber and risk of coronary heart disease: a pooled analysis of cohort studies. Arch Intern Med. 2004 Feb 23;164(4):370-6.

Stark D, van Hal S, Marriott D, Ellis J, Harkness J. Irritable bowel syndrome: a review on the role of intestinal protozoa and the importance of their detection and diagnosis. Int J Parasitol 2007 Jan:37(1):11-20. Epub 2006 Oct 12.

CHAPTER 5

The Critical Role of Gut Bacteria

This is a topic that might make some feel a little funny inside. Because, speaking of "inside," there are a lot of bacteria living in there – an estimated 100 trillion of them, 10 times more of them than there are human cells in the body. They outnumber us ten to one in our own bodies! Fortunately, the majority of them are beneficial, and they play a crucial role in our health. The bacteria in the gut work in conjunction with the colon itself. Beneficial bacteria protect the colon from the harmful bacteria, yeast and parasites that also live in the gut, and other intruders. They digest fiber to provide nutrients for the cells of the colon walls; other bacterial products help feed the liver and muscles. Colon bacteria also make several vitamins, including B-12 and K, which we can't make ourselves. The colon in turn provides a warm home for the bacteria, and its secretions help keep bad bacteria at bay.

An estimated 500 species of microorganisms live in our colons; this is often referred to as the *gut microbiome*. How did they get there, you may wonder. They've been there right from birth, particularly in the case of vaginal births. Breastfed babies achieve early colonization of gut bacteria too, but within a matter of months after birth all babies, even those born by C-section and not breastfed, acquire these bacteria from being touched and held, and from their environment.

None of us has the same collection of microorganisms or in the same ratios: each person' microbiome is as unique as they are themselves. Not only that, but an individual's lineup of gut bacteria can change from one day to the next, depending on what we eat, drugs we may take, what things we may encounter, and so on.

The makeup of the gut microbiome, as is true of any ecosystem, is in a constant state of flux or rebalancing. A 2012 study found that people who had typically eaten a vegetarian diet, and who began eating eggs and dairy products for purposes of the study, overnight had more of the kind of bacteria that tolerate bile salts, which are produced when we eat protein-rich foods. On the other hand, these particular bacteria diminished when participants switched to a carbohydrate-intense diet, and instead, there were more of the carbohydrate-handling bacteria in their guts. All the various species of bacteria have been there all along, they simply increase or decrease their numbers as necessary, in response to what we send their way. And, as might be expected, gut bacteria vary widely by a person's place of residence. Residents of the U.S. have different colonic bacteria than residents of Malawi, for example, to accommodate the variation in diet in the respective countries.

Bacteria Work Together With the Intestinal Cells

The beneficial gut microorganisms, by occupying the attachment spaces on the wall of the colon, help create a barrier to toxins entering the bloodstream; they also prevent yeast from attaching to the colon and making holes in it, which would lead to the same problem of foreign matter escaping into the blood and creating inflammation and allergies. In other words, beneficial bacteria are an indispensable part of a healthy colon, part of their function being to help prevent the damage caused by a leaky gut. Leakage of toxins into the bloodstream, the theft of vitamins by harmful gut bacteria, poor memory, anxiety, gluten intolerance, abdominal pain and food allergies are all traceable to a poor ratio of good and bad gut microorganisms. These symptoms are typical of ADHD and other conditions. The good bacteria, if sufficient in numbers, also suppress bad bacteria and prevent them from producing toxins. As well, an overabundance of bad bacteria robs us of iron, because they use it heavily in their deleterious functions; iron depletion, in turn, gives rise to metal toxicity from other heavy metals. If harmful bacteria are not kept in check by enough good bacteria, taking iron supplements or eating iron-rich foods to overcome the resulting anemia will only make the bad bacteria stronger.

Beneficial gut bacteria are also vital to our intestinal health in another way: enterocytes, the specialized cells that line the colon, have a life expectancy of only several days at most, and must be constantly replenished. Beneficial bacteria play a key role in the proper maturation of these cells. If they weren't there, the enterocytes would degenerate into mutated cells, some of them even cancerous, and would not be able to carry out their functions of breaking down and absorbing nutrients and maintaining a barrier against yeast, parasites, macromolecules and so on. This education of new gut lining cells becomes even more critical in a person undergoing chemotherapy, because fast-developing cells (enterocytes no less than cancer cells) are exactly what chemotherapy targets.

Beneficial Bacteria and the Immune System

Not only do these bacteria train the new enterocytes, they are critical to the development of the immune system. As was noted in Chapter 1, up to 80 percent of the immune system resides in the gut. An important part of that is located in the colon. Butyrate and other molecules produced by good bacteria activate macrophages in the colon to produce anti-inflammatory molecules and to help guide new T-cells to recognize which things are friends and which are foes to be attacked. Without the education brought about by the beneficial bacteria, our immune system would be much weaker. In laboratory studies, this enhancement of the immune system has been found to reduce inflammatory bowel diseases like Crohn's disease.

"Regulatory T-cells are important for the containment of excessive inflammatory responses as well as autoimmune disorders. Therefore these findings could be applicable for the prevention and treatment of inflammatory bowel disease (IBD), allergy and autoimmune disease," says Dr Hiroshi Ohno, team leader in a 2013 research project. He advocates supplying additional butyrate to the gut bacteria via the diet to enhance its immuno-protective functions. "Butyrate is natural and safe as a therapy and in addition to that it is cheap, which could reduce costs for both patients and society" he explained. In another trial, butyrate, given orally, was also proven to be an effective remedy for dysentery in a lab experiment carried out on rabbits.

The Role of Butyrate

Butyrate has been shown further to have anti-inflammatory and anti-cancer effects, and to lessen the effects of type-1 diabetes in rats. It has even been suggested that various inflammatory bowel disorders may be traced to a mere deficiency of butyrate. It is of prime importance in maintaining the integrity of the gut wall. In an experiment with laboratory rats that had been caused to develop colitis, butyrate was able to protect the gut wall from leaking. In other words, butyrate protects against leaky gut syndrome. It has been shown as well to reduce fasting insulin, and to raise insulin sensitivity by 300 percent in mice studies, along with controlling weight. This is all good news for the diabetes-prone.

Where to get this safe, natural, inexpensive miracle cure? From butter, which contains up to 4 percent butyrate (butyrate comes from the German word for butter) and aged cheese. Beneficial bacteria also make butyrate themselves in the gut, if they are supplied with fermentable fiber from our diet. Actually, it would be hard to eat enough butter and cheese to yield all the butyrate we need, so it's important to feed our bacteria fermentable fiber, also known as prebiotics. These are derived mostly from soluble fiber in such foods as sweet potatoes, oats, barley, wheat, fruits and vegetables, legumes, onion, garlic, nuts, seeds, flax seed and psyllium seed husks.

Good bacteria, and the butyrate they produce, lower the pH of the colon, i.e., make it more acid, to about 4-5 (7 being neutral). This promotes the absorption of calcium, iron and magnesium, and represses the growth of candida and bad bacteria. It also reduces the risk of colon cancer. A study published in 2014 shows that the action of beneficial bacteria, when given sufficient fermentable fiber, promotes better sugar handling, improved insulin sensitivity and even reduced fat storage and overweight in the body.

Some Benefits of a Healthy Gut Microbiome

- The good bacteria help to constantly re-establish and train the specialized cells, or enterocytes, that line the colon, which have a lifespan of only several days. Without the bacteria, they would degenerate into mutated, even cancerous cells, and could not perform their functions;

- They train new T-cells and other white blood cells to recognize which things are friends and which are foes to be attacked. Without the training brought about by the beneficial bacteria, our immune system would be much weaker;

- They lower the pH of the colon, making it more acidic, which promotes the absorption of minerals such as calcium, iron and magnesium;

- They make vitamins, including B-12 and K, which we cannot make ourselves;

- Good bacteria ferment certain kinds of fiber to make short-chain fatty acids that feed the enterocytes, and prevent bad bacteria from using the same fiber to create toxins

- They occupy attachment sites on the colon wall, preventing parasites, yeast and bad bacteria from attaching and causing damage

- They suppress yeast, preventing a candida infection and all that follows

- They help prevent colon cancer and inflammatory bowel diseases

- There is constant communication between the gut bacteria and the brain. It has been shown scientifically that our gut bacteria influence our memory and recall, and feelings of depression and anxiety as well

- They help prevent yeast from turning elemental mercury into more toxic forms

- They can chelate toxic heavy metals, holding onto them until they are passed from the body

- They have been shown to improve thinking ability and mood

A Fragile World for Beneficial Bacteria

Beneficial bacteria are obviously extremely important to our health. In fact, it has been suggested that they practically constitute another organ of the body, as essential as any other. And like any other organ, or any other good thing, there are elements that attack it. Some of the most obvious attackers are the various antibiotics that have been prescribed so freely over the course of the past decades, which wipe out beneficial flora without destroying the bad bacteria or yeast in the colon. The growth of antibiotics use has been accompanied by not only an increase in antibiotics-resistant microorganisms, but a great many diseases that were not common before. We will discuss this subject in Chapter 7. Along with antibiotics, birth control pills, steroids, chemotherapy and other drugs also kill beneficial bacteria, and we can now add to that list glyphosate.

Glyphosate is the active ingredient in Roundup, the herbicide/pesticide that is sprayed on over 90 percent of soybeans, corn, canola, sugar beets and other crops. Genetically modified crops are engineered to withstand this poison, and the poison becomes part of the plants, which carry it to the animals that eat them. It destroys the ability of plants to use certain metabolic pathways, and that feature carries on to the animals (and people) too. It binds more than 80 percent of vital minerals like iron, manganese and zinc and makes them unavailable, minerals that our tissues and enzymes must have for proper function. Many non-GMO crops, such as wheat, also are contaminated with glyphosate when it is sprayed on them to hasten ripening

Our government shows no sign of rescuing us from this chemical onslaught, much the contrary. According to Dr. Joseph Mercola, in 2013 the EPA "doubled the amount of glyphosate allowed in food... Soybean oil may now contain as much as 40 parts per million (ppm) of glyphosate. Meanwhile, research by Dr. Monika Krueger at Leipzig University shows that *a tenth of a part per million* is all that it takes to kill your *Lactobacillus, Bifidobacterium,* and *Enterococcus faecalis!* So soybean oil is now allowed to contain a whopping *400 times* the known limit at which it can impact your health."

Glyphosate is not lost in processing and not broken down by digestion. It's in probably most of our foods, unlabeled, and in our water supply. By blocking the use of essential minerals and destroying gut bacteria, glyphosate leaves us vulnerable to a whole host of modern diseases. We will discuss detoxification in Chapter 10.

Probiotics

It can be seen from the above discussion that a healthy gut microbiome is of the utmost importance to our physical and even mental and emotional health. Also, that antibiotics, birth control pills and other drugs and chemicals are the enemy of beneficial bacteria. Therefore, it behooves us to be cautious about what we take into our bodies, and to do whatever we can to build up the beneficial flora. We discussed prebiotics earlier; we also would do well to consume probiotics.

"Probiotics can improve intestinal function and maintain the integrity of the lining of the intestines," says Dr. Stefano Guandalini, professor of pediatrics and gastroenterology at the University of Chicago Medical Center. He cites evidence that probiotics are equally important for a strong immune system.

The National Institutes of Health's National Center for Complementary and Alternative Medicine (NCCAM) states in its web page on oral probiotics (accessed April 2014), that different strains of probiotics have been shown to have beneficial effects on diseases. "Strong evidence exists for acute diarrhea and antibiotic-associated diarrhea, and substantial evidence exists for atopic eczema (a skin condition most commonly seen in infants). Promising applications include childhood respiratory infections, tooth decay, nasal pathogens (bacteria harbored in the nose), gastroenteritis relapses caused by *Clostridium difficile* bacteria after antibiotic therapy, and inflammatory bowel disease." The NCCAM is looking into the benefits of probiotics on other diseases. Their medical approach focuses on the use of specific strains against specific diseases, and cautions that there is not much data available on possible long-term side effects. Obviously, there are many more conditions that would be helped by probiotics, not to mention simply our overall health – but this has not yet been "scientifically proven."

The Harvard Medical School Family Health Guide web page (accessed April 2014) says "Probiotics may also be of use in maintaining urogenital health. Like the intestinal tract, the vagina is a finely balanced ecosystem. The dominant *Lactobacilli* strains normally make it too acidic for harmful microorganisms to survive. But the system can be thrown out of balance by a number of factors, including antibiotics, spermicides, and birth control pills. Probiotic treatment that restores the balance of microflora may be helpful for such common female urogenital problems as bacterial vaginosis, yeast infection, and urinary tract infection."

A study published in 2014 demonstrated in a clinical trial that women given a strain of beneficial bacteria called *lactobacillus rhamnosus* lost more weight compared to women who were on the same diet but without this probiotic. After diet restrictions were lifted and everyone was allowed to eat whatever they wanted, the women who kept taking lactobacillus rhamnosus continued to lose weight, but the women in the control group (i.e., not taking it) gained weight. By the way, *lactobacillus rhamnosus* is the first listed type of probiotic in Young Living's Life-5 supplement. That is not to say that it is a weight-loss supplement, but it is interesting.

Probiotics for mental and emotional health

In a 2013 experiment, people who consumed a yogurt containing probiotics were compared to people who consumed a yogurt that had no probiotics and to another group that consumed no yogurt at all, as they viewed pictures of persons who were frightened or angry. It was found that those who consumed probiotics had more activity in the thinking area of the brain, as measured by MRI, than those who ate the yogurt that contained none, and that the latter group had more activity in the emotion-processing brain area. The third group showed mixed results. Thus probiotics seem to enhance thinking ability and reduce anxiety.

It is not widely known that the gastrointestinal nervous system actually produces 95 percent of our serotonin, the "feel-good" hormone, far more than the brain itself does. Indeed, serotonin is the primary neurotransmitter in the gut. So serotonin re-uptake inhibitors (prescription anti-depressants) may be causing digestive distress more than anything else – except that a 400 percent increase in autism has been found in babies whose mothers took SSRI's.

Conversely, probiotics may be an alternate treatment for depression and anxiety. According to the CDC, approximately 1 in 10 Americans were taking anti-depressants in 2011, and one in 5 women age 40-59, way too many. But in mid-2013, less than two years later, 1 in 8 Americans were on these drugs, and 1 in 4 women 50-64. With the number of people on anti-depressant meds skyrocketing in our overstressed modern society, new research is pointing us toward using probiotics to treat these emotional problems rather than drugs. In mice, at least, an experiment using *bifidobacterium longum* showed its ability to reduce symptoms of anxiety. A separate study demonstrated the ability of a *lactobacillus* strain to modulate the neurotransmitter GABA, leading to a reduction in anxiety and depression, as well as lowered levels of cortisol.

In other words, both of these types of bacteria, found in the normal gut microbiome, are capable of boosting our mood and behavior. It has also been shown that consuming probiotics (which increase helpful gut bacteria) not only boosts thinking capacity, it also improves memory formation and recall. It can be seen, then, that communication flows not only from the brain to the gut, but the other way as well, and thus that how we take care of our gut's health has a major impact on our lives as a whole. The gut has even been called the body's "second brain," and it appears the gut bacteria are a large part of that.

REFERENCES
_____

Hooper LV, Midtvedt T, Gordon JI. How host-microbial interactions shape the nutrient environment of the mammalian intestine. Annu Rev Nutr. 2002;22:283-307. Epub 2002 Apr 4

Nagendra Singh, et al. Activation of Gpr109a, Receptor for Niacin and the Commensal Metabolite Butyrate, Suppresses Colonic Inflammation and Carcinogenesis. Immunity, 2014; DOI: 10.1016/j.immuni 2013.12.007

Kennedy MJ, Volz PA. Ecology of Candida albicans gut colonization: inhibition of Candida adhesion, colonization, and dissemination from the gastrointestinal tract by bacterial antagonism. Infect Immun. 1985 Sep;49(3):654-63.

Berg RD. The indigenous gastrointestinal microflora. Trends Microbiol. 1996 Nov;4(11):430-5.

Scharlau D, et al. Mechanisms of primary cancer prevention by butyrate and other products formed during gut flora-mediated fermentation of dietary fibre. Mutat Res. 2009 Jul-Aug;682(1):39-53. doi: 10.1016/j.mrrev.2009.04.001. Epub 2009 Apr 19.

Canny GO, McCormick BA. Bacteria in the Intestine, Helpful Residents or Enemies from Within? Infect. Immun. August 2008 vol. 76 no. 8 3360-3373

The Importance of Fermentable Fiber http://www.prebiotin.com/fermentable-fiber/#sthash.MidmTBkW.dpuf

Lupton JR. Microbial degradation products influence colon cancer risk: the butyrate controversy. J Nutr. 2004;134(2):479-482.

De Vadder F, Kovatcheva-Datchary P, et al. Microbiota-Generated Metabolites Promote Metabolic Benefits via Gut-Brain Neural Circuits. Cell - 16 January 2014 (Vol. 156, Issue 1, pp. 84-96)

Kanauchi O, Iwanaga T, et al. Butyrate from bacterial fermentation of germinated barley foodstuff preserves intestinal barrier function in experimental colitis in the rat model. J Gastroenterol Hepatol. 1999 Sep;14(9):880-8.

Zhanguo Gao, Jun Yin, Jin Zhang, Robert E. Ward, Roy J. Martin, Michael Lefevre, William T. Cefalu, and Jianping Ye. Butyrate Improves Insulin Sensitivity and Increases Energy Expenditure in Mice. Diabetes. Jul 2009; 58(7): 1509–1517. Published online Apr 14, 2009. doi: 10.2337/db08-1637 PMCID: PMC2699871

Verena J, Koller VJ, et. al. Cytotoxic and DNA-damaging properties of glyphosate and Roundup in human-derived buccal epithelial cells. Arch Toxicol. 2012 Feb 14. Epub 2012 Feb 14. PMID:22331240

Samsel A, Seneff S.Glyphosate's Suppression of Cytochrome P450 Enzymes and Amino Acid Biosynthesis by the Gut Microbiome: Pathways to Modern Diseases. Entropy 2013, 15(4), 1416-1463; doi:10.3390/e15041416

Heimen, Julius Genetic Engineering: the Glyphosate threat http://www.rag.org.au/modifiedfoods/rounduphealthissues.htm

Samsel A, Seneff S. Glyphosate, pathways to modern diseases II: Celiac sprue and gluten intolerance. Interdiscip Toxicol. 2013; Vol. 6(4): 159–184. doi:10.2478/intox-2013-0026

CHAPTER 6

The Kidney: Murky Mere or Crystal Clear
(WINTER - PART I)

I find it interesting that the kidney is cleansed before the liver in the natural, annual energy flow of the body. If you remember, the colon gets its energy in the fall, the kidney in the winter and the liver in the spring. The reason the kidney comes second, after the colon, is that the kidney is the next most important eliminator in the body. It filters the blood and sends minerals and electrolytes back to the body and toxins and blood-borne wastes to the bladder as urine. If the kidney isn't up to speed, when you go to do a liver cleanse, and if the colon isn't clean, you can become fairly sick as you retain the toxins that were dumped by the liver, couldn't get through the colon and were resorbed into the circulation, and then weren't eliminated from the body by the kidney. So it matters that we do everything in order.

Each kidney has about one million nephrons that enable your two kidneys to filter approximately 17 pints of blood every hour. These nephrons can become destroyed or blocked by disease processes or other means. One of the major ways the kidney can become blocked is through the formation of stones. Kidney stones can be formed from calcium, phosphorous, oxalic acid or uric acid. If the kidney is failing to filter out excessive uric acid, a by-product of undigested proteins, gout can result. If the digestive tract isn't working right, or if a person is taking the wrong kind of calcium, (calcium citrate and calcium lactate are the ones you want) calcium deposits can occur anywhere in the body in the form of spurs, osteoarthritis, soft-tissue deposits, kidney stones, etc.

Kidney stones

A huge contributor to phosphoric stones in the body is carbonated drinks (soda pop). Not only do the phosphates contained in the soda contribute to the formation of stones, but they also may leach calcium from the bones, leading to osteoporosis. Cola drinks, coffee, tea and other caffeine drinks may actually leach more fluids from the body than they provide, according the University of Maryland Medical Center. In addition, they decrease the amount of citrate in the body, and citrate is a stone inhibitor since it binds with calcium and draws it out of the kidney. Some research shows that drinking one quart (less than three 12-ounce cans) of soda per week may increase a person's risk of developing stones by 15 percent. One kidney specialist commented that he would be out of business without soft drinks. Of course, the effects are not always immediate or universal, so many people may cheat disease for years.

Another consideration in stone development is the acidity of the urine. A diet high in proteins not only contributes to gout but also to higher urine acidity, not to mention an over-acid body in general. The average human being really requires only 2 ounces of protein per day to replace what is used up by the body. That's just half a quarter-pounder! Excess sugar or carbohydrate intake can also cause increased urine acidity. Why should you care about acidic urine? Because in addition to causing discomfort upon urination, a high acid environment promotes formation of kidney stones. It also causes osteoporosis as the body draws calcium from the bones to try to buffer the excess acidity.

Kidneys need water

Probably the single greatest cause of kidney malfunction or destruction is insufficient water intake. The kidney needs plenty of water to perform its job. A 150-pound person should be drinking eight 8-ounce glasses of water a day as a bare minimum for the body to function properly, including adequately flushing the kidneys. Some sources say one quart per 50 pounds of body weight is the minimum. Within reason, more is better. The kidneys don't mind having plenty of water; they can deal with lots of water more easily than too little. This means pure, filtered water, not juice, milk, soda or other drinks. These do bring some water into the body, but it is bound to some degree to the solutes in the liquid and, as discussed above with regard to caffeinated drinks, some may actually pull water from the body rather than supplying it. Way back in Charles

Dickens' day it was noted that soft drinks left people more thirsty than they were before drinking them.

Poor hydration causes the blood and lymph to be thick and sluggish and may lead to blood pressure problems, urinary tract infections, and the accumulation of stones and toxins in the kidney that do not get flushed out. Many times people become dehydrated because they find it inconvenient to have to stop what they are doing and use the bathroom, or perhaps they are out in public and don't want to use the public restrooms, so they don't drink enough water. This is not good for the kidney nor the body in general. When the body can't void, toxins accumulate, resulting in nausea and headaches, and the body will be forced to send the excess toxins either to the liver to be processed or to other tissues to be stored to remove them from circulation.

Many years ago, my husband was hospitalized with a kidney stone. After 5 days of lying in a hospital bed with strong drugs to control the pain, he passed the stone, only to have the very same thing happen with the other kidney a few months later. It was not pleasant! He then began drinking 3 liters of water daily, and within a matter of weeks felt smaller stones flushing out of his kidneys on their own. He never had another kidney stone attack. Moral of the story one more time: drink plenty of water.

When a person has a sharp pain in the mid back, the first thing he or she should do is grab a glass of water. Most times it is just a signal that they are dehydrated and the kidney is calling for more water. A sharp pain in the mid back or flank right below the ribs could also mean a person has a kidney infection or kidney stones. However, simply drinking a gallon of water in a day's time and also drinking a few quarts of cranberry juice or taking a high-quality concentrated cranberry supplement will many times take care of it. However, if the pain continues you should get immediate medical attention; stones can be excruciatingly painful (as mentioned above) if ignored to the point they cause an attack, and kidney infections can be extremely serious. The kidney is such an important organ you must not neglect it.

Helpful measures

We have had a lot of success flushing kidney stones using Idaho Balsam Fir oil. This oil seems to dilate the ureter and allow the stone to pass. Other essential oils that help with stones are Geranium, Valor and Juniper. It really helps when dealing with kidney pain to make a compress of 3 drops each of

Rosemary, Sage, Juniper and Idaho Balsam Fir. Place the oils in a bowl of hot water, soak it up with a small towel, and put the towel across the back over the painful kidney. Leave it there for 30 minutes or more. Repeat as needed.

K&B tincture is helpful for any kidney pain or infection or simply as a tonic to strengthen the kidneys.

Valor is an extremely helpful essential oil for the kidney. The reason for this probably is that kidneys hold the emotion *fear* and Valor is formulated to help combat fear. Just putting 6 drops of Valor on the kidney acupressure/reflex points on the sole of each foot (see Appendix A) once a day does wonders for the kidneys and the body in general. One of my patients stated that after three months of putting 2 drops of Valor on her feet 3 times daily to help her get rid of panic attacks, her kidneys started to drain and she lost 35 pounds in water weight over the course of just a few days. Several months later, she was again under stress so she put soaked a cotton ball with Valor and slipped it just under her blouse where she could smell it all day. She said the oil acted like a natural diuretic and she again drained a lot of excess water.

The following remedies for kidney stones from The Essential Oils Desk Reference have been excellent for passing or dissolving kidney stones and clearing out the kidney. I alternated each drink every hour during one severe bout of kidney stones.

Kidney Stone Drink #1

5 drops Rosemary
5 drops Geranium
5 drops Juniper
1 Tbs agave nectar
  (I used real maple syrup)

Juice from ½ lemon
8 oz. warm distilled water.

Mix together, shake well and drink on an empty stomach 2-3 times daily until the stone passes.

Kidney Stone Drink #2

2 Tbs. virgin olive oil
8 oz. organic apple juice

Mix vigorously and drink; repeat 2-3 times daily until stone passes.

In addition to filtering the blood and its other functions, the kidney is the major regulator of blood pressure in the body. Its job is to measure the sodium and potassium balance of the blood. If one or the other is out of balance the kidney will send a signal through a complicated pathway to constrict or dilate the blood vessels thus raising or lowering the blood pressure.

High blood pressure/hypertension

One of the most frequently asked questions I get is: "What one oil can I use to lower my blood pressure?"

I get that "what one oil can I use" question a lot, abut all kinds of things. First, there isn't one oil for any one symptom. It is a symptom, after all, not a cause of your difficulty, and there can be many causes for the same symptom. High blood pressure is a symptom. Pain is a symptom. Headache, stuffy nose, cough, aching joints, blurry vision, mental fog, dizziness, are all symptoms that could have different causes. Moreover, different causes need different essential oils.

Since high blood pressure is closely tied to kidney function, I decided to discuss it here in the kidney chapter.

High blood pressure—also known as hypertension— increases the risk for heart attack, stroke, kidney failure, coronary heart disease, and other serious health problems. Blood pressure is the force of blood pushing against the inside walls of arteries. The harder your heart pumps and the narrower your arteries are, the higher your blood pressure rises. Over time, the wear and tear caused by untreated high blood pressure can damage your blood vessels and vital organs.

Stress

The Number 1 cause of high blood pressure is stress or tension. The stress you feel may even include past stresses or emotional stresses that have not been handled. Therefore, meditation and energy or emotional work would be in order here. In the 1970's scientific research proved that the best thing to reduce blood pressure was biofeedback. That research was not highly publicized, since it didn't lead to a profit-making drug. Biofeedback can include, for example, the person going into meditation and imagining that their blood pressure is normal. I know that meditation itself is extremely restful giving the body the rest it needs.

If you are feeling stressed, support the adrenals with Super B, Mineral Essence and OmegaGize[3], Nutmeg essential oil, Clove essential oil or EndoFlex essential oil blend. Feeding the adrenals is important, as the adrenal gland needs these nutrients daily to make hormones for the body and to produce energy, and stress burns through them. CortiStop Women's Capsules are fantastic for reducing stress and I have seen it reduce hypertension. Use the Feeling Kits by Young Living oils to let go of past traumas.

The Peace and Calming and Valor blends help a person relax. B vitamins, calcium and magnesium are important in supporting the nervous system.

Increasing these nutrients will help a person manage his or her stress level. Exercise and recreation can also help a person relax. A good hot bath in Epsom salts and Peace and Calming essential oil blend is another excellent relaxant. So is a good massage or a Raindrop Technique. Some doctors recommend cutting back on salt intake. It may also be a good idea to increase your potassium intake to help balance the excess salt we typically consume, often unknowingly, every day. Bananas and apricots are an excellent source of potassium.

Kidney problems

The 2nd cause of high blood pressure is kidney problems, as they are in charge of dilating or constricting the veins and arteries to regulate the pressure. So clean and support the kidney. You can clean it by doing a Master Cleanse. Using Young Living's K & B formula along with Juniper, Sage, and Rosemary essential oils support the Kidney in its functions.

Lungs

The 3rd cause of High BP is lung difficulties. The kidney sends a signal to the lungs to make the hormone produce Angiotensin II that dilates and constricts the veins and arteries. If this is not being done correctly or if the Lungs have some disease it can cause high BP.

Breathe deeply into the lungs Raven or Ravintsara to assist the lungs in making that hormone. (If the liver is not functioning right then the body won't have building blocks to make that hormone.) Of course quitting smoking will greatly improve lung function. Harmony oil blend has been a great help for some to stop addictions to smoking. Smell it when you wish you could have a cigarette.

Other causes of high blood pressure

The 4th cause of high blood pressure is blockages in the veins and arteries. The liver could contribute indirectly to high blood pressure if it isn't digesting either fats or proteins or both. A liver cleanse to assist the liver in digesting fats, proteins and calcium, along with Essentialzymes-4 between meals to digest the excess fats, proteins and calcium in the blood and in the veins and arteries would be essential here. See Chapter 9 of this book.

The 5th cause of high blood pressure is heart problems, according to conventional medicine, but the super drug of the day is not the best way to treat them. Garlic and vitamin E not only support the heart but also help to lower blood pressure. Use Aroma Life to assist the heart. There are a number of ways to use essential oils to assist the heart; see pages 7 and 24 of my book Ultimate Balance to learn more.

If high blood pressure is a problem for you, it would be advisable to get a medical exam to discover the cause. A Complete Blood Count (CBC) should be a part of the exam, as well as a cholesterol panel to check for any underlying problem with cholesterol handling. If there is a cholesterol problem, consider liver enzymes and cleansing to help the liver enhance its capacity to digest fats and regain control over cholesterol levels (see chapter 7).

Important! Low blood pressure often stems from under-hydration rather than from an organic kidney problem. Try drinking more water!

Even if you aren't having kidney problems it doesn't hurt to simply take K&B tincture, and use Juniper, Geranium and Valor essential oil blends around the first of January every year just to help clean and clear the kidney in general. Rub the Valor on the kidney reflex points of the foot, and take a drop or two each of the Geranium and Juniper oils in a glass of water two or three times a day to flush the kidneys.

The University of Maryland Medical Center posted the following on their official website (unfortunately, it has since been removed) and it contains excellent recommendations for maintaining good kidney health:

◆ Drink more water
◆ Reduce salt intake
◆ Reduce protein intake
◆ Increase calcium citrate or lactate
◆ Increase vitamin B6.
◆ Increase fiber-rich foods and their compounds
◆ Increase essential fatty acids including fish oil
◆ Decrease purine-rich foods (for people at risk for uric acid stones). These include beer and other alcoholic beverages, anchovies, sardines, organ meats (e.g., liver, kidneys), legumes (e.g., dried beans, peas, and soybeans), mushrooms, spinach, asparagus, cauliflower, and poultry.

Case History

Mark was brought to my office by his parents. Mark was 80 pounds oveweight and was quite chunky for a nine-year old boy. His skin was tight around his face, hands, arms, legs and feet. I examined him and determined tht he had water weight gain. His stomach just sloshed back and forth with all the excess water in it. His parents informed me that they had seen a medical doctor who had given him a diagnosis of idiopathic nephritis and told them that the kidneys were being destroyed and that the boy probably wouldn't live past the age of 13. They said that it was a rare condition and that there was nothing that they could do.

I explained to his parents that idiopathic meant that there was no known cause and that the doctors couldn't figure out a cure. I put my head to it for a few minutes pondering what would cause the kidney to dump so much water into the surrounding tissues. I thought about mineral, salt and sugar imbalances. Then suddenly, I had a strange thought, one that would make the medical doctors laugh at me and tell the parents that I was a quack. The thought was "holes." I thought about large holes that would allow proteins to leak out of the kidney, causing water to be drawn osmotically into the tissues to dilute the proteins. "what would cause such holes?" I pondered. Suddenly I thought of worms and wondered whether he had a parasite destroying his kidney.

This was in the early days of my using essential oils so I didn't have all the tools that I now have. I put him on rectal injections of Parafree. I also put him on Valor essential oil blend and Juniper essential oil I knew that Valor when used heavily can act as a diuretic. I also knew that Juniper was specific for the healing of the kidney. Three months later, Mark and his parents returned. I didn't even recognize him. In front of me was a normal-sized nin year old boy. Mark's parents said they had taken him back to the medical doctor, who was amazed at what had happened and asked what had caused such a change. They told him about my treatment, and sure enough, the doctor told them I was a nut and quack. I suppose his opinion could be disregarded since the treatment worked! I saw Mark last year, a healthy, wiry, 15 yea old boy. His parents told me that he had never had any more kidney problems.

Note: I saw Mark again in 2014, and he was still thriving at 22 years of age.

CHAPTER 7

Yeast Infection: Surprisingly Deadly
(W I N T E R - P A R T I I)

Yeast (*candida albicans*) grows naturally in the colon and is harmless and possibly beneficial in small amounts. It seems to help control the bad bacteria there. It exists on the outside of the body as well as the inside, along with innumerable species of bacteria. They are part of our world. However, sometimes we can get an overgrowth of yeast in the colon, often as the result of excessive use of antibiotics, which kill bacteria but not yeast. Unfortunately, antibiotics will indiscriminately kill the friendly bacteria in the colon as well as the target bacteria that purportedly caused some disease or another.

As discussed in Chapter 4, the friendly bacteria or flora that live symbiotically in our colons are important for a number of reasons, but most significantly for this particular chapter, they keep the harmful bacteria and yeast population under control. When there are not enough friendly bacteria in the colon to control the yeast present there, we get out-of-control yeast growth, causing the body to be flooded with the mycotoxins and alcohol the yeast produces, giving rise to potentially severe mental, emotional and physical problems, as serious and unexpected as Multiple Sclerosis, for example.

One of the ways friendly bacteria keep yeast under control is by maintaining a slightly acidic environment in the gut. Yeast as well as other bad actors require an neutral to alkaline environment to flourish. Without beneficial bacteria and their acidic secretions to keep it in check, yeast will morph from an ovoid, budding shape to a malignant rhyzoid network of spiky, tubular shaped fungi (aka hyphae, or micelia), and will act to alkalize the gut even more by excreting ammonia gas so as to create conditions that promote faster multiplication. In this form it creates dozens and dozens of toxins (up to 79 by some counts) and also creates holes in the colon wall, allowing macromolecules of foreign matter and undigested proteins to enter the blood system, leading to allergies and diseases. Here is another motivation to keep your colon clean: so that if for some reason you kill the beneficial bacteria with antibiotics, the perforation of the colon by runaway candida will not allow toxic impacted fecal matter to leak into the bloodstream.

If left unchecked, candida can spread from the colon throughout the body. Blood temperature is ideal for candida, as is blood pH. If candidiasis progresses far enough, it will aggressively insinuate itself into your cells and organs and make itself part of them, just as mold (another fungus) can become part of the very fabric of a basket of forgotten damp laundry. Fungi attack organic matter. Not to put too fine a point on it, with the beneficial gut flora wiped out, the candida fungus thinks you are dead too and is trying to decompose you!

Symptoms of Candidiasis

Dr. William Crooks, in his book "The Yeast Connection," describes over 450 different symptoms of yeast overgrowth. These include such symptoms as irritable bowel syndrome, vaginal infection, hormonal imbalance, chronic sinusitis, fungal growths on the skin or nails, thrush in the mouth, headache, fatigue, mood swings, depression, suicidal thoughts, slow learning, brain fog, memory problems, inability to concentrate, allergies and decreased immune system function.

These symptoms can give you a good idea whether you have a yeast infection. But apart from symptoms (which you may not identify as stemming from yeast), if you have been on antibiotics for any length of time, or had chemotherapy, or are taking steroids, antacids, ulcer medications or birth control pills, you have created the conditions for a yeast overgrowth and probably have one. Excess sugar consumption, so common in our modern diet, also has a lot to do with yeast overgrowth, since sugar is the favorite food of yeast. The yeast population can potentially double in two hours in a warm environment, as in the colon, with the right amount of sugar, and then can keep increasing exponentially to the limits of available food. To make things even worse, the alcohol that a rapid growth of yeast produces is detrimental to friendly bacteria. A "sweet tooth" probably stems from the candida itself demanding that you feed it the sugary food it needs.

Dangers of Candidiasis

Candida is the leading cause of mortality from infection introduced by catheters.

Candida has been shown to convert mercury to a methylated form that is stored in body fat, and is much more difficult to get rid of.

Candidiasis is a very serious condition and may be at the root of a great many named diseases that are typically diagnosed and treated individually – even cancer. It is found in as many as 91 percent of ulcerative colitis cases alone, and has likewise been associated with Crohn's disease, irritable bowel syndrome (IBS), rheumatoid arthritis, asthma, excema, hives, peptic ulcers, lupus, depression, personality changes, schizophrenia, autism and ADHD. In this masquerade, you may never succeed in healing from those other diseases that you supposedly have, because what you really have is candidiasis.

Dr. William Shaw of Great Plains Laboratories blames tartaric acid created by candida for most of these diseases, and states that he has seen more than a thousand cases of autism reversed by anti-fungal treatment. He also says that this same tartaric acid is the culprit in chronic fatigue, fibromyalgia and muscle weakness, through its interference with the Krebs cycle, which is the primary way cells create energy. Other candida mycotoxins cause additional ailments.

Dr. T. Simoncini, among others, sees a direct connection between candida and cancer. These doctors say that every tumor removed is covered in candida. Dr. Simoncini says, in fact, that in his experience, cancer *is* candida!

The medical establishment is skeptical about candida and reluctant to diagnosis it except as an oral or vaginal infection – until an immuno-compromised patient dies of it, and it is discovered in autopsy. To be fair, doctors are under a lot of pressure to make quick diagnoses so they can code their findings and be paid by the insurance companies, whereas candidiasis is difficult to diagnosis and routine lab tests are of no help in identifying it. So your best chance of enjoying good health includes being aware, yourself, of the many manifestations of candida and how to deal with it.

Candida test

There is a simple test you can do yourself for candida, as follows: First thing in the morning, before you eat or drink anything, even water, take a clear glass of water, work up some saliva and spit it into the glass. Check it every 15 minutes for an hour. If it remains a blob on top of the water, you probably don't have candida. On the other hand, if the spittle spreads out, develops long tendrils hanging down, sinks to the bottom of the glass or creates specks in the middle of the water, you very likely are infected with oral candida at the least. But your symptoms and history may be the best guide.

Prescription and over-the-counter remedies are available, but I do not recommend them. They can cause liver and kidney damage, and migraines as well, and once they are discontinued the yeast comes back with a vengeance. Further, yeast learns to produce a biofilm to protect itself from the pharmaceuticals that are meant to kill them, and they soon become ineffective. Yeast is very adaptive and resilient. I believe natural methods are more effective than pharmaceuticals, don't create resistance and are much easier on the body. If you use natural methods to control yeast you will very likely have the flu-like symptoms of yeast die-off, but you won't have the side effects and after-effects of pharmaceutical drugs.

Again, even if a pharmaceutical drug is able to kill off a systemic yeast infection, yeast will come right back! It's all around us in the environment and will re-infest us one way or another and begin to grow again inside, unless it is kept under control by the gut microbiome.

Dealing with Candida

One "natural" way of clearing yeast overgrowth that has been widely used over the past 20 years or so has been to take 15 garlic pills and 15 acidophilus pills a day, decreasing over a period of three weeks to 5 of each per day, and then staying at that level for 2-3 years until the yeast is all gone. Other herbs to support the body during this time would be caprilic acid, pau d'arco, yellow dock and immune-building herbs such as cat's claw (uña de gato).

There are other effective, natural ways to deal with yeast that take much less time. There are two aspects to an effective protocol for taming yeast. The first is diet modification to starve the candida so it cannot continue multiplying. The second is to reduce it to its proper balance in relation to good bacteria, which is a very small ratio.

If you have been diagnosed with a yeast infection or suspect one based on your own self-observations and you want to get rid of it, let me emphasize from the very beginning that you <u>must</u> follow a strict diet while working to get rid of yeast. If you don't, you may render useless any other processes at work on the problem. This is true, in fact, with regard to almost any disorder, disease, or dysfunction. Good food can help us keep our body's own natural disease-fighting system, the immune system, in top shape, while helping us feel better and live longer. On the other hand, unwholesome foods and unnatural products can, over a long or even short period of time, reduce the immune system's ability to fight disease as well as keep our bodies from functioning at their best. Refined sugar is one of the worst stressors of the immune system and, as it happens, is also the favorite food of yeast.

A colon cleanse will help with cleaning out the yeast and possibly other parasites that have moved in while the colon has not been functioning properly. Doing a colon cleanse first, before going on the yeast diet will allow the dead yeast organisms to be eliminated from the body more easily, and will help to decrease the toxic reaction, sometimes called a healing crisis or Herxheimer reaction, that is often associated with yeast die-off. Alternatively, it is also helpful to do a Master Cleanse first to clear the way.

Be sure to use probiotics, including acidophilus and bifidus, to fill the space of the yeast that has died. Take them from the beginning of your candida cleanse. These friendly bacteria will take control of the microbiotic environment of the colon so that the yeast won't be able to come back as a problem. A good quality yogurt containing a variety of live cultures will help re-establish the right balance in the colon. You will have to buy a top-notch name brand yogurt to be sure of getting sufficient high-quality live cultures. Some cheap "yogurts" have no probiotics in them at all. Kefir is even better for you than yogurt, and you can make both of them at home yourself for best results. But at first you would do well to take a more concentrated source of probiotics in capsule form. Capsules can contain billions of helpful bacteria versus the millions available in yogurt. Life-5 from Young Living is an excellent probiotic. (Life-5 replaced the discontinued Royaldophilus.)

The diet

The diet for fighting yeast overgrowth is as follows: For the first two weeks eat only meat and vegetables, with the exception of such vegetables as potatoes, peas, sweet potatoes and sweet corn (which is not really a vegetable anyway). These vegetables are high in starch, a substance the body quickly processes into sugar, which feeds yeast. Remember, sugar is the main enemy when trying to control yeast. In this diet, meats are considered to include all the usual meats, poultry and fish, plus eggs and nuts (walnuts, pecans, almonds, cashews, etc. and their nut butters). Some exclude peanuts (technically they're legumes) from the list because they may carry mold from growing underground.

Fats do not promote yeast growth, so they are not restricted in this diet. In fact, coconut oil has been shown to kill yeast in lab experiments, so it's definitely something to include in your anti-candida diet.

Sauerkraut and <u>raw</u> apple cider vinegar are great additions to the diet; fermented foods are full of probiotics that feed beneficial bacteria. For the best results, ferment your own vegetables! Please note that there are different kinds of fermentation; they're not all one and the same. The yeast that can turn into candida is not the same as yeast as in grain or the bacteria in fermented vegetables.

Drink only water. No carbonated beverages, ever (no, not even if they are sugar-free). It should go without saying that you cannot drink alcoholic beverages. No breads, grains, cakes, sugars (including honey, molasses, corn syrup, high-fructose corn syrup, maple syrup, cane sugar, beet sugar, all-fruit jelly, fresh or dried fruits or fruit juices etc.). Please don't replace them with artificial sweeteners, which may not feed candida but are quite detrimental to your health for other reasons. Milk and milk products and anything containing these as ingredients are likewise not allowed. In this diet tomatoes are considered a vegetable, and corn is considered a grain, so you can eat tomatoes but not corn.

You may be aware that our brains and cells use glucose for energy, and worry that sugar restriction is hazardous for that reason. Not to worry, you can derive glucose from the yeast cleansing diet, and besides, your brain and other cells can also use fats for energy. But no *trans* fats please!

Here are the foods that are allowed or forbidden during the yeast cleanse, in list form:

Allowed

- Meat
- Fish
- Eggs
- Nuts (except peanuts)
- Vegetables, including fermented vegetables (except those on the forbidden list below)
- Fats (coconut oil is preferred)

Forbidden

- Sugar in any form (glucose, maltose, fructose, anything ending in -ose)
- Carbonated beverages
- Milk
- Fruit and fruit juice
- Grains and flour
- Sweet corn
- Potatoes
- Sweet potatoes
- Peas

Ways to Boost Your Cleanse

While you are on the strict anti-yeast diet, I highly recommend you add the following remedies for faster results than you would get with diet modification alone or with the standard garlic-acidophilus-herbal approach:

1) Melrose, (an oil blend produced by Young Living Essential Oils); it contains one of the strongest available forms of tea tree oil (melaleuca), a proven yeast killer. Take 25 drops of Melrose in a capsule 3x a day. Another way of using Melrose is to put 15 drops of it in one cup of cold water and use this as a retention enema (hold for 15 minutes) every few days. You may find enemas unpleasant, but this clears up candida in a matter of weeks versus years of using the garlic capsule method. Even better is to mix 15 drops of Melrose into a quarter cup of coconut oil, put it in a syringe and use that as a retention enema. You will need to cool the filled syringe first so that the mixture is a semi-solid and doesn't come right back out. This should be done just before you go to bed, to prevent too much leakage.

2) Other powerful candida-fighting oils include Thyme, Patchouli and Cedarwood. Clove and Lemongrass have been demonstrated to also inhibit the creation of protective biofilm by the candida organism, which makes them especially useful. Be cautious in using Clove, Lemongrass, and Thyme, though; they are very hot oils. Put only 7 drops in coconut oil, and use it as a retention enema.

3) For small children put 1-4 drops of Melrose into a capsule and put it in a spoon of peanut butter or applesauce to help the child swallow the capsule. Do this three times a day. Many people just use the Melrose plain in the child's mouth or put 3 drops in an eye dropper and insert it into the rectum twice a day.

4) Stevia (available at supermarkets or health food stores) is also very effective in killing yeast. Take 2-3 drops by mouth 3 times a day. Stevia will also give a sweet taste in your mouth, for a change from meat and vegetables.

Doing all of the above, instead of the garlic routine, should take care of mild vaginal yeast infections in a matter of a day or so, and will get rid of major colonic or systemic infections with months or even weeks. Although this protocol does not seem to include anything directly targeting systemic candida, the Melrose in particular will spread from the colon to the rest of the body to attack the fungus wherever it is. Again, a rigorous diet is indispensable for best results. Yeast is a fierce opponent and will fight hard to survive. Don't be easy on it!

Stay on this meat and vegetable diet conscientiously for two weeks, and then begin reintroducing a single, simple food to your diet every four days. The reason for adding foods one at a time is that yeast cleansing changes the colon and its digestive processes. Some foods, when introduced back into your diet, might cause stomachache, headache, vomiting, diarrhea, gas, a rash or other symptoms. These may in fact be foods to which your body has always been sensitive ("allergic") without your realizing it. By introducing or reintroducing foods one at a time, you can see which one causes a problem. It also lets your enzymes ramp up slowly. If you have a reaction to a food, avoid it for a month or two before trying it again.

Start by adding in the grains. Rice and quinoa are the mildest grains and rarely cause reactions. Add one or the other to your diet, and eat it as often as you want for 4 days. Hopefully you will be able to eat it without a problem. Wheat often causes a reaction because of the way it is abused in processing, so be careful with it. It goes without saying that highly refined grains are far from what nature intended. In fact, I suggest you begin with sourdough bread (the real stuff from a bakery, not sourdough-flavored supermarket bread) or learn to make your own, because it's much easier to digest. After the grains, try various fruits. Be aware that fruits and milk too will often cause reactions. Once you have tried simple foods, you can experiment with more complex foods.

Stay away from white sugar, forever—it feeds yeast, plays havoc with your blood sugar levels, adds calories without giving you any vitamins or minerals at all, and weakens your immune system. High-fructose corn syrup is even worse. Instead, cook with stevia, fruits, fruit juice and honey as sweeteners. Molasses has a strong taste that not everyone enjoys but, on the plus side, it does contain iron and other minerals. If you absolutely must use sugar, at least make sure it is dehydrated cane juice or raw cane sugar. Dates are an excellent way to sweeten things. Also avoid supermarket milk if at all possible. Pasteurized, homogenized milk is not good for you—with or without BST – but raw milk is fine.

Increasing your mineral intake can help with the killing of yeast. Yeast dies in the presence of copper. However, because copper and zinc compete for the same receptor sites we don't want to put too much copper into our system—it could lead to a deficiency of zinc. One way to get copper is to leave a washed and clean penny overnight in either lemon juice or vinegar. Then use the lemon juice or vinegar any way you normally do. Be careful not to overdose on copper as it can increase the body's stress reactions. Buckwheat is a good source of copper, as is barley grass juice. But whole barley, eaten as a grain, may exacerbate gluten tolerance problems in certain individuals. To avoid this problem, grow your own barley grass, cut it at 3-4 inches high and juice it. There is no gluten in the green blades, only in the grain. Alfalfa juice is another good green drink for copper intake.

Quite often when killing yeast you will have a die-off reaction as mentioned above, sometime between day three and day ten. You may feel achy and sick. You might have a severe headache, mucus secretions or feel like your bones are going to break or even have emotional disturbances. If this happens, add blood purifiers to help. Yellow dock and red clover help, as do lemon enemas. The oil blends I generally recommend to help with clearing toxins from the blood are Juva Cleanse and Purification. I recommend 1 drop by mouth every minute for ten minutes, then 1 drop every 10 minutes until the reaction stops and you feel better. Epsom salt baths and soaking in a warm tub with several drops of Clove oil also will pull toxins. Just relax and soak for 15-30 minutes. Some of the symptoms of die-off are caused by acetylaldehyde. You can help your body break it down by taking molybdenum and iron.

Here again is a list of the recommended products that kill yeast and aid in recovery:

Melrose oil blend
Clove, Lemongrass, Thyme, Cedarwood, Pachouli essential oils
Stevia
Juva Flex and/or Purification oil blends
Clove oil
Epsom salts
Coconut oil
Life-5 (contains acidophilus and other probiotics)
VerdiSyn or Perfect Food
Mineral Essence (contains molybdenum and iron)

REFERENCES

Crook, William G., The Yeast Connection: A Medical Breakthrough. Random House. New York, NY. 1986

Trowbridge, John P., MD., and Dr. Morton Walker. The Yeast Syndrome. Bantam Books. New York, NY. 1986

Randolph, Theron G., MD. and Ralph W. Moss Ph.D., An Alternative Approach to Allergies. Harper &Row. New York, NY.1989

Martin, Jeanne Marie. Complete Candida Yeast Guidebook. Prima Publishing. CA. 2000

Essential Desk Reference, Essential Science Publishing USA 2001

Hidalgo, Jose A., and Jose A. Vazquez. "Candidiasis." eMedicine. Eds. David H. Shepp, et al. 14 Jul. 2008. Medscape. 3 Nov. 2009 <http://emedicine.medscape.com/article/213853-overview >.

Bergsson G, Arnfinnsson J et al. In Vitro Killing of Candida albicans by Fatty Acids and Monoglycerides. Antimicrob. Agents Chemother. 2001, 45(11):3209.

Staniszewska M, Bondaryk M, Siennicka K, Kurzatkowski W. Ultrastructure of Candida albicans pleomorphic forms: phase-contrast microscopy, scanning and transmission electron microscopy. Pol J Microbiol. 2012;61(2):129-35.

Sudbery, Peter E.. "Growth of Candida albicans hyphae". Nature Reviews Microbiology 9 (10): 737–748.

Lacour M, et al. The pathogenetic significance of intestinal Candida colonization: A systematic review from an interdisciplinary and environmental medical point of view. International Journal of Hygiene and Environmental Health. 2002;205:257

Douglas LJ. Candida biofilms and their role in infection. Trends in Microbiology. Jan 2003; 11 (1): 30-36. DOI: 10.1016/S0966-842X(02)00002-1.

Shaw, William, The Yeast Problem & Bacteria Byproducts http://www.greatplainslaboratory.com/home/eng/candida.asp

Kaufmann, Doug, The Fungus Link, MediaTrition, Rock Wall TX, 2008.

Crump, J. A., and P. J. Collignon. 2000. Intravascular catheter-associated infections. Eur. J. Clin. Microbiol. Infect. Dis. 19:1-8.

Mohd Sajjad, Ahmad Khan, Iqbal Ahmad. Biofilm inhibition by Cymbopogon citratus and Syzygium aromaticum essential oils in the strains of Candida albicans. Journal of Ethnopharmacology. 27 Mar 2012; 140 (2): 416-423. DOI: 10.1016/j.jep.2012.01.045.

Abe S, et al. Anti-Candida albicans activity of essential oils including Lemongrass (Cymbopogon citratus) oil and its component, citral..Japanese Journal of Medical Mycology. 2003; 44 (4): 285-291.PMID:14615795

Simoncini, Dr. T., Cancer is a Fungus, Edizioni; 2nd edition (September 1, 2007) 245 pp

CHAPTER 8

The Master Cleanse and More
(WINTER - PART III)

After completing the colon cleanse, followed by a kidney cleanse and, if necessary, going through a parasite cleanse and/or a yeast cleanse, you are ready to start the Master Cleanse originated by Stanley Burroughs. It is sometimes referred to as the Lemonade cleanse. The booklet written by Stanley Burroughs on the Master Cleanse is available from Life Science Publishing.

As the name implies, it has a cleansing and rejuvenating effect on most of the organs of the body. Completing the colon, kidney and parasite cleanses puts the body in a condition to gain maximum effect from the Master Cleanse.

I like to do the Master Cleanse before a liver cleanse since it helps to eliminate a lot of toxins before you get into the heavier cleanse of the liver. You should also be having <u>at least</u> one, preferably two, good bowel movement a day before you start the Master Cleanse. Less than that could result in a toxin build up that might make you ill. The Master Cleanse is not a liver cleanse *per se*, but rather a total tissue cleanse. It changes the pH of the body and helps not only to clean out the liver but also pulls toxins from other organs, muscles, joints, lymph and skin, and flushes out mucus. It also cleans up insulin receptor sites on cells, diminishing insulin resistance, which is great news for diabetics.

Stanley Burroughs came up with this cleanse before essential oils were widely available to the public. He believed that one shouldn't take any nutritional supplements nor any other support while on the cleanse. However, in using the Master Cleanse in my practice, I have found that essential oils and other Young Living products help make this cleanse more effective. Therefore in writing this chapter I have included the oils that to increase the effectiveness of this cleanse.

I have also noted problems that some of my patients encountered while on this cleanse and the ways we found to deal with those problems. This chapter has excerpts taken from Healing for the Age of Enlightenment by Stanley Burroughs, available through Life Science Publishing. To completely understand how this cleanse works I suggest you read his book.

The Master Cleanse consists basically of a salt water flush in the morning followed by a lemonade fast the rest of the day, and no other food. As a preparation to make the beginning of the cleanse more comfortable, the evening before you start the cleanse, take a drop or two of Peppermint oil along with one or two capsules of Comfortone and 1 tablespoon of ICP. In the morning begin with the salt water flush.

Salt Water Flush:

To do the morning salt water flush, add 2 level teaspoons of non-iodized sea salt to a quart of lukewarm water. Mix well, then drink the entire quart. Yes, this can be a little challenging, but you need to drink the entire quart in order to get the right results. Try to drink the salt water within 15 minutes. It's also a good idea to massage the colon. Make sure you use *non-iodized* sea salt, because regular iodized salt will not have the same beneficial effect and may overload your system with iodine. This oral enema will flush out your entire digestive tract, including the colon, from top to bottom. This will usually happen within 30-60 minutes, prompting you to eliminate 2-4 times, clearing out the plaque and debris from the walls of the digestive tract as well as the parasites that have been living there.

If diarrhea is a problem during the flush, it helps to use ½ tsp to 1 Tbs of ICP at night to better form the stool. Some people get severe diarrhea with the salt water drink, which makes it awkward if they have to work. The ICP will help prevent that.

Burroughs recommends that you start every day of the cleanse with this drink. If you are having extremely runny stools, this could lead to a mineral imbalance followed by serious complications and you will need to use Mineral Essence to help correct the problem. In an emergency, if you don't have Mineral Essence at hand, you can use an electrolyte drink. A mineral imbalance manifests itself in several ways. One is that the body will buzz like pins and needles, sometimes in the extremities and other times in the face or all over the body. Another symptom of a mineral deficiency could be increased stress or depression or suicidal thoughts. (This could also stem from not drinking enough of the lemonade drink described below.)

If you feel that drinking the salt water every day is too hard on you, take a good laxative tea or use Comfortone and Peppermint oil every night to ensure that you have a healthy bowel movement daily, and take the salt water flush on alternate days. But do not skip the salt water altogether or the cleanse will not be as effective. The salt water helps remove the toxins and other debris from the entire digestive tract, as stated above. Some people complain of nausea after drinking the salt water. A drop of Peppermint oil will help clear that up. You can either take it by mouth or rub it on your stomach area.

After the salt water flush each morning, you can begin drinking the maple syrup lemonade.

Maple Syrup Lemonade:

You'll need, per glass:

- 2 tablespoons fresh-squeezed lemon juice (approx. 1/2 lemon)
- 2 tablespoons pure maple syrup, Grade B or Grade C (the darker the better), organic if you can find it
- 1/10 tablespoon cayenne pepper to start, gradually increased during the course of the cleanse (the more BTUs the better)
- 10-14 oz pure water

Mix together and drink 8-12 glasses daily.

Do not use bottled lemon juice. Freshly squeezed lemon juice is alkaline but begins to get acidic in just a few hours. For this reason it is best to make only as much lemon juice as you can drink at a time. Some people like to squeeze enough lemons for the entire day's drink since they need to take it to work. They then measure out 2 tablespoons at a time. Burroughs says that this is fine as long as you don't add the water to it until you are ready to drink it. I have noticed, however, that it still changes taste by evening and is a little more acidic by then.

Do not use pancake syrup. It is best to use grade B (or C, if available) maple syrup. The darker the maple syrup the more minerals and nutrients it has, and this is what is going to sustain you as you are cleansing. Grade A syrup is over-refined and lacks the minerals required to feed the body while on this cleanse. Pancake syrup is NOT maple syrup. It is usually simply corn syrup with imitation maple flavoring. It has no nutritional value whatsoever and, unlike real maple syrup, has a very high glycemic index. Don't use it.

The maple syrup feeds the body, the lemon juice alkalizes the body, and the cayenne pepper helps circulation, artery and vein dilation and is a catalyst for chemical changes in the body, including helping the cells to excrete toxins. If you have a hard time with the cayenne pepper, start with a tiny pinch and increase the amount every few days until you can handle the heat. We have found that taking cayenne pepper in capsules or leaving it out of the drink noticeably reduces the chemical reactions in the body and the cleanse is not as effective. Be brave!

No Substitutions, Please

As a side note, I once had a patient who came in and claimed that the Master Cleanse didn't work at all for her. I inquired further and found out that she didn't have fresh lemons so she used bottled, concentrated lemon juice; she didn't have maple syrup so she used either plain table sugar or honey; and she didn't have cayenne pepper so she used Tabasco sauce! Of course the Master Cleanse didn't work for her—she was never on it!

Drink the lemonade at least every 2 hours. It is important to drink 8-12 10 oz glasses of lemonade a day. Drinking less than this can cause severe headaches, hunger or hypoglycemia along with depression or suicidal thoughts. Eat no other food. The lemonade contains all the minerals and calories necessary to sustain the body. If you get hungry or dizzy or experience headaches, mood changes, depression or sudden anger, drink more lemonade! Your blood sugar has dropped and you are not drinking enough of it or else you are not drinking it frequently enough.

The Master Cleanse has become popular among celebrities as a method of slimming down for a film or a public appearance, rather than maintaining a healthy lifestyle. Sometimes people get overexcited because of the sudden weight loss that can occur on this cleanse and they think that if they drink less lemonade they will lose even more weight. This is not healthy for you. The Master Cleanse is not intended to be a weight loss diet; it is intended to get rid of toxins. Most people I know who have been on the cleanse gain their weight back in a short period of time after completing it. Meanwhile, the lemonade is your only source of nutrition: Don't short yourself.

If you are hypoglycemic before you start this cleanse you can still do it, but be sure to drink plenty of lemonade. If you are diabetic you should substitute molasses for the maple syrup as it will not raise your blood sugar as rapidly, but still contains minerals and nutrients. Some people with hypoglycemia have had success using a scoop of Powermeal a day in addition to the lemonade. I would recommend just trying to drink more lemonade if you feel hypoglycemic symptoms (dizziness, severe hunger, headache, depression, anger, sudden drowsiness.)

As mentioned earlier I like to use Comfortone and ICP while on the Master Cleanse. The reason for this is that Comfortone contains bentonite clay and other herbal colon cleansers that help absorb toxins from the colon. The bentonite clay helps loosen and remove plaque from the walls of the intestines. The ICP helps form a stool to keep you from being too loose and also acts like a big brush to remove old debris. I also like to take Essentialzyme as it helps to break up plaque and mucus.

Herbal Laxative:

Burroughs recommends that each evening right before bed time you drink an herbal laxative tea to help with elimination. You can use senna tea or peppermint tea for a laxative. A drop or two of Peppermint oil in the mouth along with a capsule or two of Comfortone also work well as a laxative in place of these teas.

Trouble shooting:

In addition to the problems listed above, many people get headaches while on the Master Cleanse. This is to be expected the first few days as the cleanse starts at the top of the body, works it way down, and then works from the inside or core out to the extremities. After about 3 days the headaches should subside. Don't forget that one cause of headaches may be not getting enough of the lemonade drink. Another cause may be that so many toxins are being released from the body rapidly. If you have headaches the first few days it helps to use essential oils for relief. Peppermint, Wintergreen, Panaway, Juvaflex, Purification and Juvacleanse are some good oils and blends to use to help relieve the headache. Purification helps clean out the toxins in the blood if taken by mouth a few drops at time. Take one drop a minute for a few minutes until the headache is relieved. For general aches and pains of the body, soak in Epsom salts combined with a few drops of Clove oil in the tub. That also helps remove toxins from the body. Using a total body detoxification machine such as the EB-305 or the B.E.F.E. machine will help to remove unwanted toxins also.

Going Off the Lemonade Fast

Burroughs recommends a minimum of 10 days on this cleanse. He suggests that you stay on it until the white coating on the tongue disappears. I have known many people who have gone 40 days on the Master Cleanse and loved it. However, for some people it was more difficult. They preferred doing the cleanse once a week every month for several months. To go off the cleanse after having been on it for several days or more, it is important to follow the next instructions carefully. The body has not had food to digest for several days and giving it food suddenly can make you sick and cause your digestive tract to not work properly. First Day: Start with 4 oz. fresh-squeezed orange juice mixed with 4 oz. water. If it goes well, drink several more 8 oz. glasses of fresh orange juice during the day. Sip slowly. Dilute with water if needed. Continue drinking the lemonade between times. Second Day: Drink several 8 oz. glasses of fresh-squeezed orange juice during the day-- with extra water, if needed. The lemonade drink is still your source of nutrition.

In the evening of the second day make a vegetable broth. Make it fresh; no canned soup. Use seasonal leafy and root vegetables such as beets, beet tops, turnips, turnip greens, kale, carrots, onions, parsley, celery, potatoes, okra, one or two kinds of legumes, squash, beans, a little salt, cayenne pepper and dehydrated vegetables, some of these or as many as you can find. Cook lightly. Drink the broth, eating only a few bites of the vegetables. Third Day: Orange juice in the morning. At noon have some more of the soup you made with some of the vegetables. No meat, fish, eggs, bread, pastries, milk, tea, or coffee. For dinner, have the vegetables from the soup. Fourth Day: Orange juice or lemon and maple syrup in the morning. Fruits, vegetables, seeds, nuts for lunch. Have salad or fruit for dinner. Fifth Day: Eat normally but no junk food, dairy, tea, coffee, white flour or white rice or heavy animal proteins. If, after eating is resumed, distress or gas occurs, go back to the lemonade diet for a few days until the system is ready for food.

Some people have complained of getting gall stones immediately after the Master Cleanse. If you have pain in the upper right quadrant of the abdomen, it might be gall stones or it might be a clogged cisterna chyli, which is a less serious condition. Go back on the lemon cleanse immediately. Use warm compresses of Ledum, Juva Cleanse and Juva Flex and take these oils internally. It would be wise to see a doctor to make sure that you don't have a stuck gall stone.

I have seen fantastic results with the Master Cleanse but as you can see from this chapter there some problems that might arise. It would be wise if you are going to go on this cleanse to do so under the supervision of a natural healthcare doctor who can help you with any of the physiological problems that might come up.

Lose Fat, Lose Toxins

While doing the Master Cleanse many people tend to slim down, as noted above. Although the Master Cleanse is not intended as a weight-loss program, it is an opportunity to rid ourselves of some of the toxins that were stored in the body fat you are dropping. (That is where the liver hides away the toxins it cannot deal with, to get them out of circulation.) As long as we are letting go of fat, we can be pro-active in helping flush those toxins out of the body. Many of these toxins can be eliminated through the skin, the body's largest organ, by sweating. Here are my suggestions:

First, find a time during the morning to do all of the following steps:

1. Take 3 Super-B capsules all at once. This will cause heat and itching due to the niacin. When that happens, it means toxins are being released, and you are ready for the next step.

2. Exercise for 10 minutes to get your heart rate up and the blood flowing well so that the toxins are mobilized.

3. Drink 1-2 drops of Peppermint oil in a cup of warm water

4. Soak in a bathtub with 7-10 drops of Peppermint oil pre-mixed with a cup of Epsom salts, in water as warm as you can comfortably stand. You may want to agitate the water from time to time to keep the oil from floating on top while you are soaking.

5. As soon as you begin sweating, time 15-20 minutes longer to stay in the tub. Have water nearby to drink if you need it. If you should feel light-headed before the time is up, you may need to cool the water just a bit. A drink of Ningxia Red and a dose of trace minerals will help too.

6. You will probably itch after you are finished. Wash off with a half and half blend of vinegar and water, or shower.

7. Take calcium, sodium, potassium and magnesium as well as trace minerals to replace what you lost by this procedure.

The niacin in the Super B's mobilizes the fat and the heat created by the Peppermint and the hot bath cause the toxins to sweat out through the skin.

Some of the toxins that are being flushed may be drug residues or metals. To help deal with the problems of getting these and other toxins out of the body via the bloodstream, take methionine. Also, take activated charcoal or bentonite clay to capture them as they are dumped into the intestines by the liver, so they can be carried out and eliminated.

I would advise doing this sweat detox once or twice a week. Do it in the morning so you have time to recover before you go to bed. It is a great way to get rid of fat-stored toxins, and it may be done while simply dieting too, as calorie restriction will mobilize fat as your energy supply, thus releasing those toxins for you to flush out.

CHAPTER 9

The Liver: Your Body's Chemical Plant
(SPRING)

The liver is an extremely important organ of the body and if not working properly can give rise to a wide range of physical AND mental problems. The liver handles over 50,000 chemical functions. It cleans and filters the blood. It is in charge of metabolizing fats, sugars and proteins. It clears toxins from the body. It breaks down drugs and other chemicals. It produces enzymes to help digest food, and bile to help emulsify and absorb fats. It produces and regulates cholesterol. It regulates hormones and hormone production.

It balances sugars. For the most part anyone who is having mild to severe sugar handling problems, including diabetes mellitus Type II and hypoglycemia, should look first to the liver as the source of their problems as the liver is the major sugar handler of the body. Anyone with a hormonal imbalance should look to the liver because it is the major hormone balancer. Most of the time, hormone imbalances result from the liver not digesting fats properly to create the building blocks from which hormones are made.

Anyone who has a lot of allergies, especially spring and fall hay fever and sensitivities to chemicals, would be well advised to do a liver cleanse, because as much as 90 percent of allergies will begin to clear up after a colon and liver cleanse!

Anyone who seems to have a weak immune system is probably not metabolizing (in the liver) the proteins needed to make white blood cells, so once again it would be wise to do a liver cleanse.

As can be seen, a well-functioning liver is a major factor in an individual's overall health.

The liver's woes

There are many causes of liver congestion and malfunction. Eating a poor, unbalanced diet either too high in carbohydrates or too high in protein can cause liver congestion. It is well known that excessive consumption of alcohol destroys the liver, and so does acetaminophen. (Acetaminophen is even used purposefully in scientific research to destroy liver tissue.) Other over-the-counter drugs and prescription medications can exhaust or even damage the liver. The same goes for recreational drugs and vaccinations.

The bottom line is that the liver must deal with almost every toxin that enters the body—even those that could potentially kill it!

The liver can also be overtaxed by overeating, even with good food, or with too much nutritional supplementation and too many minerals! I had a young patient, actually only 3 years old, whose mother had put her on a mineral supplement that included colloidal silver, and she was on it for about a year at an adult dosage. Her skin had become gray from excess silver. Fortunately, it completely cleared up after a few months of liver cleansing.

In addition to the many harmful things we ingest purposefully, are all the things we inadvertently take into our bodies every day, it then being the liver's responsibility to get them out again (if it can). These include such things as gasoline fumes when we fill our gas tanks, exhaust from cars and trucks, outgassing from carpets and drapes and pressed-wood products, toxic fumes and chemical compounds in soaps, shampoos and detergents, household cleaning products, smoke from various sources and other forms of air pollution, and of course all the food additives of various kinds, on top of the pesticides and herbicides sprayed on plants in the field. Then there are the hormones that have been fed to the animals whose meat we consume—the liver has to isolate them, break them all down and get rid of them. It's a tough job being a liver in these modern times.

Enzymes are an important part of a liver program. Taking the right kind of enzymes will take some of the load off the liver. Even after a liver cleanse, it is wise to continue to take enzymes because our manufactured foods these days are stripped of them.

The following is a list of the some of the problems you might experience if your liver is functioning at a less than optimum level:

- Over weight, or inability to lose weight
- Abdominal bloating after eating, excess gas
- Poor/ inadequate digestion
- Frequent or continued fatigue
- Mental fatigue
- Frequent headaches or migraines
- Mood and behavior swings
- Clinical depression
- Bad breath
- Coated tongue when going without food for a half or full day
- Irritable bowel syndrome
- Sluggish metabolism
- Over-burdened, weakened immune system
- High cholesterol
- Excessive body heat
- Gallbladder problems

- High blood pressure
- Sugar cravings
- Sugar imbalances
- Hormonal imbalance
- Oily skin
- Skin blemishes, discoloration, acne, psoriasis, warts, moles, or generalized itching rashes
- Intolerance to chemicals
- Intolerance to smells
- Allergies, both food and chemical
- Diminished eyesight
- Heartburn or acid reflux
- Low sex drive, impotence
- Sleep disorders
- Poor protein utilization
- Anger and irritability
- Gall stones
- Poor memory
- Premature aging and graying

It was discovered in 1995 that the liver could completely regenerate itself. That's great news. Amazingly, when two-thirds of a liver is removed in surgical experiments, it will grow back to full size often in as little as a week, and if transplanted will adjust its size, whether larger or smaller, to the size of the recipient. But a sick liver can't regenerate itself very well—it has all it can handle just trying to keep going. Thus the need to cleanse it.

Cleansing the liver

It takes time to cleanse the liver. As the liver dumps its toxins through the blood they will recycle several times through the liver before they are completely removed from the body. Pharmacists understand this about the liver and note what is called the half-life of a drug. This refers to how much of the drug gets detoxified through the liver each round until there is so little it does not have an effect on the body anymore. Research has shown that the liver will encase some of these toxins in fat and store it either in the liver or in the tissues themselves.

Burdock and yellow dock herbs have a long history of use as liver cleansers. These herbs are effective, however it takes months and sometimes years to completely cleanse the liver using herbs alone. Using these herbs yearly is an excellent way to keep the liver clean for someone who is not having a lot of problems with liver toxicity. Unfortunately, we are living in an ever more toxic world.

Fasting is one of the best ways to heal and clean the liver. If we could do a total fast from all foods and pollutants of every kind for a period of 40 days, the rested liver probably would completely heal itself. However, since that obviously is not possible, we can rest the liver with frequent, less-extreme fasts.

The Master Cleanse is a good liquid fast to rest the liver. Some cultures fast 24 hours, with complete abstinence from foods and liquids to rest the body, once a month. Others fast 10 days in the spring and again in the fall, but rather than abstain completely from food and drink, these cultures do juice fasting. Juice fasting is a great way to rest and cleanse the liver.

Carrot juice has long been known as an excellent liver cleanse. Because of its high glycemic index, carrot juice is often mixed with other juices such as spinach, apple or beet juice. Carrot and beet juice are an excellent combination for cleansing the liver. Carrots have also been employed to purify and revitalize the blood. They are rich in minerals and beta carotene that will support and rebuild the liver. Carrot juice has often been called the "the miracle juice." My first introduction to natural healing was in 1981 when I met a woman who drank carrot juice daily. She claimed that she had overcome many of her health problems just through drinking carrot juice. Unfortunately, I was not ready to leave the Western medical model at the time, and drinking raw carrot juice seemed strange. But had I embraced only carrot juicing and nothing else way back then I could have saved years of ill health.

A toxic and damaged liver reduces its capacity to store vitamin A. Without vitamin A inflammations and infections begin to attack skin and surface membrane of all mucous and serous membranes. Vitamin A protects the integrity of these tissues. Inflammation and infection is the beginning stage of many chronic diseases. Dr. Bernard Jensen says that "Because so many of the problems resulting from a Vitamin A deficiency are accompanied by a sluggish, toxic or hypoactive liver, we must consider the easiest assimilable form of this vitamin under such conditions. Carrot juice is the best choice at present." He further states that carrot juice is rich in carotene which is assimilated much more easily than vitamin A from fish oils or organ meats. He claims that carotene in large doses is not toxic to the body like vitamin A itself can be, and that the body easily converts carotene, a nutrient found in abundance in the yellow and orange vegetables, to vitamin A.

Beet juice is probably one of the best of all vegetables juices due to its high mineral content. Not only is beet juice good for liver ailments such as jaundice but it is also excellent for the gallbladder and the kidneys. Beet juice reportedly will dissolve calcium deposits in the body and is excellent for the veins, arteries and bones.

Coffee enemas are also touted as being able to clean the liver. I have never personally done a coffee enema nor had a patient do one, though I have heard many doctors say that if you are drinking coffee, you are putting it in the wrong end!

I followed a beet/carrot juicing program for four straight months after I had a severe bout with poison ivy that I had inadvertently swallowed, which caused my internal organs, especially the liver, to swell. Thanks to the carrot and beet juice, the swelling in my liver gradually decreased and it returned to normal. I noticed during that time that the hay fever I had once had came back while my liver was acting up, but as I followed the juicing program the hay fever went away again.

Before you attempt a liver cleanse you need to cleanse your colon so the toxins released from the liver will be able to exit the body and not get stuck. My advice is to take it slow and easy on this one. DO NOT start the liver cleanse until some other cleansing is done first. Instead, begin with a colon cleanse as outlined in Chapter 4, then the kidney cleanse (Chapter 5).

Then, if necessary, do a yeast cleanse (Chapter 6.) Follow that with the Master Cleanse (chapter 7), which is a whole-body cleanse, including another cleanse of the colon.

The ideas behind a liver cleanse

After you have done the Master Cleanse for at least 10 days in a row your body is prepared to do a liver cleanse. Starting on a liver cleanse before completing the Master Cleanse or at least a colon cleanse could cause real discomfort as the toxins that have been stored in the liver will circulate through the blood before being eliminated. I advise that you stay on Comfortone and ICP or a bentonite clay and charcoal product while doing a liver cleanse as they will bind with the toxins that are released and assist in removing them from the body.

The basic idea of a liver cleanse is to rest the liver and let it cleanse and heal itself by going on a juice fast or at the very least eating foods that are easy to digest and healing to the liver. These foods include raw fruits and vegetables, especially dark green leafy vegetables. I also recommend that you choose at least one fruit or vegetable from each color daily. There are red, orange, green, yellow, and purple or blue fruits and vegetables. Each color of fruit or vegetable contains different vitamins and minerals that build different body systems. For example, yellow fruits and vegetables act as laxatives and tonics, while the green vegetables are rejuvenators, being rich in chlorophyll, a great blood builder. Choose also plants that have a high mineral content like turnips, beets, sweet potatoes and carrots. All the root crops are high in minerals.

Eating raw or juiced fruits and vegetables will not only give you vitamins and minerals that might have been destroyed in cooking or processing, but will also supply needed enzymes that will help digest the food and will also assist the body in getting rid of chemicals and toxins. Enzymes use minerals in their chemical reactions so choosing fruits and vegetables with high mineral content will boost enzyme function. Enzymes are an important part of a liver program because a good enzyme supplement will take some of the load off the liver. Even after a liver cleanse, it is wise to continue to take enzymes because our manufactured foods these days are devoid of them.

Don't forget the contribution that the leafy vegetables make to the body by not only supplying fiber that carries toxins out but also supplying B vitamins that help the nerves and muscles to function properly. Thirty to forty percent of the diet should consist of raw fruits and vegetables. Remember that raw fruits and vegetables also contain anti-cancer phytonutrients.

Your diet should include essential fatty acids. These key nutrients are found in cold pressed oils, nuts, seeds, avocadoes, and fish. The omega 3 and

6 oils have anti-inflammatory properties and assist the immune system in its inflammatory response. In addition, fatty acids are building blocks to hormones and feed the brain. The liver, as has been said, is a fat handler. Greasy fats or trans fatty acids such as those found animal fats, fried foods, processed foods, junk foods or processed vegetable oils that contain hydrogenated fats or rancid fats it create a high workload for the liver and gall bladder. The liver will store some unnatural fats, leading to obesity and heart diseases. These greasy fats not only clog the arteries and veins but also contribute to one of the leading causes of liver failure, fatty liver. Eating the healthful fats noted above will keep the liver and the body running smoothly. Healthful oils include flax seed oil, evening primose oil, black current seed oil and fish oils. Olive oil is also excellent for health. Choose unrefined, cold-pressed oils. One good rule of thumb is to take a teaspoon of a good oil with every meal. This will not only give your body the right kind of oil that it needs but it will also keep you from over-eating—sometimes we just keep eating because the body is searching for missing nutrients, like the right kind of fatty acids, and doesn't give us the signal to stop.

It's a good idea to think as "natural" as possible. Stay away from artificial chemicals and toxins such as insecticides, pesticides, and artificial sweeteners and colorings, flavorings and preservatives. Avoid alcohol. Alcohol leads to all kinds of liver diseases. Cut down on over-the-counter medications of any kind. Research is now showing more and more the effects of even seemingly mild drugs on the kidney, liver and heart.

Another principle to remember about good liver health is the balance of food that you eat. The body only recognizes three food groups: proteins, carbohydrates and fats. Proteins come from meat, eggs, legumes, and nuts. Carbohydrates come from fruits, vegetables and grains. Fats come from nuts, animal fats, butter, creams, oils, etc. Many diet books recommend that every meal should consist of 70% carbohydrates, 20% protein and 10% good fats, but it's important that those carbohydrates be primarily from whole, raw foods. When you eat too many carbohydrates in the form of simple sugars, breads, starches or desserts, the liver has to convert those sugars to fat. Eating a balanced diet helps keep the insulin and glucagon hormones in balance with one another and the liver functioning optimally.

Liver cleanse protocols

So what do we do to clean up the liver?

I suggest you follow one or the other of the following two protocols. The first one is simple but will take more time to completely cleanse the liver.

- Take one JuvaTone pill the first day, adding one pill a day until you get to 5, then keep taking 5 a day for the duration of the cleanse.
- Use 3- 15 drops of Juva Cleanse a day or as needed. (I usually do 3 drops 5 times a day.) "As needed" means for nausea, headaches, stomachaches, gas, aches and pains, etc.
- Stay on this protocol for 4 months, then begin noticing whether your symptoms have gone away. It will probably take longer than 4 months, perhaps up to 18 months.

The second protocol is my favorite. It does take more effort, because you have to make two juices to drink, but it works faster. Drinking these cleansing juices while also taking the Young Living products is easier on the body and makes for a quicker, effective cleanse. I felt better on it, had more energy and had a quicker cleanse. With the juices, the JuvaTone, Juva Cleanse and other supplements, it only takes 4-6 months to clean a liver, whereas the first protocol, above, may take 18 months. You can do modified juicing if you prefer, just drinking the juice a few times a day instead of every hour. That is still effective.

This cleansing protocol is called the Re-JUVA-nate diet. It has been updated a little from the original to incorporate the new products that have been introduced since the time of the first one, and also includes Vital Life juice. Here's how it goes:

- Immediately after you wake up: Drink a 10 oz glass of the special lemonade drink (the recipe is given the daily schedule):
- And take these supplements:
  2 JuvaTone
  2 Detoxzyme
  2 Essentialzyme-4
  20 Drops of Juva Cleanse in a capsule (or in a tsp of some nutritious oil, or if you choose to take it directly by mouth, i.e., by applying it to your inner cheek, you only need 3-4 drops 3 times a day.)

- One hour later, drink the Vita Life juice (the recipe is given below, following the lemonade recipe):
- Alternate the lemonade drink with Vita Life juice every hour throughout the day.
- For lunch eat a salad with 1 tablespoon Juva Power mixed in.
- Drink a glass of Powermeal sometime during the day to sustain you.
- For dinner eat a light meal. Salads, nuts, sprouts, sweet potatoes, nuts, or nut butter, fish or a small amount of poultry, fresh natural grains like quinoa, millet or brown rice and some flaxseed or cod-liver oil are wonderful to keep the liver cleansing. Avoid pork and pork products and fatty red meats.
- And take the same supplements as in the morning:
  2 JuvaTone
  2 Detoxzyme
  2 Essentialzyme-4
  20 Drops of Juva Cleanse in a capsule (or in a tsp of some nutritious oil.)

This is an amazing and powerful Liver Cleanse. Make sure you are still having 2 or 3 bowel movements a day, like you started having with the colon cleanse, to get the toxins released by this cleanse safely out of the body. If you aren't still having 2-3 bowel movements a day, take ICP and Comfortone as directed in Chapter 4 to get back to that condition.

Lemonade drink recipe:
　　2 Tbl fresh squeezed lemon juice
　　2 Tbl grade B maple syrup
　　10 oz purified water
　　1/8 tsp cayenne pepper

Vital Life juice recipe:
　　3oz beet
　　1oz celery
　　1oz carrot
　　1/3 oz Black Spanish radish (or Daigon Radish or White Radish)
　　1/8th oz ginger root
　　1/3 oz red potato

Just as a side note, some people complain that Juva Cleanse is a bit pricey, so I would like to explain what is in it that makes Gary Young like it so much, and makes it so effective.

1) Ledum acts as an enzyme, digesting toxic waste in the liver and breaking down fat molecules where toxic substances have been stored.

2) Helichrysum chelates metals and chemicals. French research has shown that Helichrysum dilates the liver ducts and facilitates the release of toxins and poisons from the system. Ledum and Helichrysum work together to break down and let go of the toxins.

3) Celery seed purges the liver as a natural diuretic for the liver. It helps transport away the toxins that are being released.

4) Carrot seed, along with Helichrysum, dilates the bile ducts to allow all this toxicity to easily exit the liver and gallbladder.

Be sure you sip your juice drinks slowly and don't gulp them down. Gulping down any vegetable or fruit juice can lead to a plunge in blood sugar. If you find that happening to you after drinking fresh fruit or vegetable juice, take an ounce of NingXia Red juice to help stabilize the blood sugar.

Both of these juice drinks need to be made fresh each time if at all possible. Admittedly, it can be difficult to juice vegetables at work. If you do not have access to a refrigerator where you can keep your juice at your workplace it may be impossible even to take juice with you. In that case the best you can do is to drink as much juice as possible in the morning before you go to work and again in the evening when you come home. I recommend you start drinking beet/carrot juice as soon as the vegetables become available in the spring and continue on through the summer until fall. To be assured of getting the best carrots and beets, grow your own in peat moss and compost. They can easily be grown in pots or placed in flower gardens around the yard.

Remember that in any fast where there might be a lot of water loss it is important to take a mineral supplement to keep the electrolytes balanced.

If you choose to take yellow dock along with the other aids, take 6 capsules a day.

It is possible to do the liver cleanse before you do the Master Cleanse if you simply feel you have to, but it is taxing on the body because as the liver dumps its toxins, if they can't quickly exit the body you can experience flu-like symptoms—aches and pains, nausea, headache and bone aches. As I have frequently pointed out, it is better have the body prepared to let the toxins flow freely out of the body.

To help ease the symptoms in the event you do cleanse too fast you can soak in 1-2 cups of Epsom salts and 5-10 drops of Clove oil in a bathtub full of water. (Clove is a 'hot' oil so it is wise to add it to 2 tablespoons of bath gel or bath salts before putting it in the tub.) DRINK LOTS OF WATER.

Peppermint and Purification oils are other options you can use. Peppermint oil will help with cramps, gas or other stomach pains, and Purification oil will help clear the blood of toxins and ease any aches and pains. Another palliative measure you can take if you feel too toxic while cleansing the liver, is to take Detoxzyme or Allerzyme between meals; they contain additional herbs and nutrients that absorb toxins from the blood.

Some people do not need to follow such a strict liver cleanse regimen, although I think it would help anyone to do so. As stated earlier it would be an excellent thing to do each spring, as soon as you can get fresh organic carrots and beets. It will not only cleanse the liver but the lighter, healthier food will also ease the energy burden on the body as it prepares for the hotter months. You'll feel better!

Case History

In early December I got a cold. It progressed and turned into what I thought was bronchitis as my lungs really hurt, especially on my left side. I even went to our family physician, who was open to natural healing. He suggested a few things that I wasn't already doing, so I added a few more supplements to the oils and other supplements I was already using. As Christmas drew nearer I became more tired and run-down and the deep cough I had developed began to really hurt my chest, to the point that the pain was almost unbearable on my left side.

The pain in my left chest continued to get worse, even though it only hurt when I coughed, which was now infrequently. Dr. LeAnne Deardeuff, my dear friend who lived many states away, encouraged me to get it checked out. So the day before Christmas, I went to my Chiropractic Physician, Dr. Christopher Gouse in Enola, PA. He was concerned I had something serious going on in my lungs and insisted I get chest x-rays taken. I did, but they showed nothing that would cause the pain. Dr. Gouse then insisted

I get an MRI of the chest. He said the pain did not seem normal and that an MRI would show things the x-ray did not. We scheduled the MRI for a few days after Christmas.

The MRI was a first for me. The dye they put in by injection burned terribly and the itching seemed to stay with me all day. The MRI was an experience I will always remember. I wondered how I had gotten to this situation and wondered what was going in my body that I thought had done such a good job to take care of. I reflected on how I had been so careful about my diet when I first started into natural healing, but now I would "cheat" every now and then and have some things I knew weren't good for me.

The MRI results were surprising. The radiologist explained that all the pain I was having was caused by a tiny cyst or tumor on the top of the left side of my liver. As I coughed, my diaphragm would push down and put pressure on the cyst. The doctor's suggestion was to just wait and do nothing. He said the cyst was too small to remove, but if I waited it would continue to grow and eventually I would be able to have surgery to remove it and see whether it was cancerous or exactly what it was. I thought that was the funniest thing I'd ever heard of! Wait? Then have surgery? Was he joking? I knew exactly what I needed to do!

When I arrived home that day I got out my Re-JUVA-nate Your Health booklet by D. Gary Young and looked at the pictures of livers. There was mine on page 8! Cystic Liver was listed as being "caused by cumulative DNA damage resulting from excess lipid peroxidation and lack of dietary antioxidants." Well, there was the solution! I would cleanse my liver as I'd already been taught by Gary and start drinking Berry Young Juice (now NingXia Red) faithfully!

The Liver Cleanse program as outlined in the book wasn't as hard as I expected. I learned to <u>love</u> JuvaPower. My body said "Thank you" every time I drank it. I even learned to like the Vital Life juice. To help with the cost of the JuvaCleanse oil (I was to take 20 drops in a capsule according to the booklet) Dr. LeAnne suggested I take fewer drops but directly in my mouth. Although it wasn't my favorite taste, that is what I did. As I started the program, it was really amazing. Within a week my pain was gone! Everyone asked me when I would have the follow-up MRI the radiologist said I would need to see if the growth was gone. I didn't want to put any more chemicals in my body and felt I already had my answer. The pain was gone and I felt soooo much better! I stayed on the program for about a month.

For maintenance now I begin daily with half a lemon, in 10 oz of water with a little agave. I also have JuvaPower and Power Meal frequently. I take Detoxyzyme, JuvaTone, ICP, Lipozyme and on occasion, JuvaCleanse oil and several other Young Living supplements and oils. And of course I have my daily dose of NingXia Red. If I am feeling sluggish or start to feel tired or that I might be coming down with something, I treat myself to three or four ounces of NingXia Red! Using Berg's table in the Re-JUVA-nate booklet, I am mindful of foods that are acid binding or acid forming and am more true to myself with what I should and shouldn't eat. I won't say I haven't ever fallen off the wagon and succumbed to something I shouldn't have, but as a rule, I am faithful to what I have learned and give my body what it really needs. My body in return serves me well!

Quin Stringham
Carlisle, PA
August 29, 2006

REFERENCES

Guyton, Arthur C. Textbook of Medical Physiology. W.B. Saunders Company. Philadelphia PA. 1991

Drugs & Liver Damage, HepCnet Hepatitis C Resources & Support, http://www.hepcnet. net/drugsandliverdamage.html

Beers, Mark H., M.D., and Robert Berkow, M.D., The Merck Manual, Merck and Co., Inc. 2005 17th Edition Sec 4 Chapter 43 Drugs and the Liver

Worman, Howard J., M. D., The Liver Disorders Sourcebook, Columbia University, New York, NY 1999

Cabot, Sandra, MD, The Liver and Detoxification, http://www.liverdoctor.com/02_ liverdetox.asp

Randolph, Theron G., MD. and Ralph W. Moss Ph.D., An Alternative Approach to Allergies. Harper &Row. New York, NY.1989

Liver Health Articles, American Liver Foundation, http://www.liverfoundation.org/db-select/articles/CatLivInj/1/1/ascend/Validated

Reducing Indoor Air Pollution, California Air Resources Board, http://www.arb.ca.gov/research/indoor/rediap.htm

Kowalchik & Hylton, Rodale's Illustrated Encyclopedia of Herbs, Rodale Press, Emmaus PA, 1987

Pedersen, Mark. Nutritional Herbology, Pedersen Publishing. Bountiful UT 1988

Keith, Velma J. and Monteen Gordon, The How To Herb Book. Mayfield Publications, Pleasant Grove UT 1989

Jensen, Bernard, D.C. Food Healing For Man, Bernard Jensen Publishing 1983

Carper, Jean. The Food Pharmacy. Bantam Books, New York 1988

Nutrition Table, Beetroot, http://flavoursofindia.tripod.com/beetroot.html

Nutrition Table, Carrot, http://flavoursofindia.tripod.com/carrot.html

Walker, N.W., Raw Vegetable Juices: What's Missing in Your Body. Health Research, 2003

Sears, Barry, PhD, A Week in the Zone. Regan Books, New York 2000

CHAPTER 10

Metals and More: Modern Hazards

One of the perils to our general health that we face in our times, that was not an issue previously, is heavy metal pollution. Heavy metals are not the same as the metals our bodies are designed to use in metabolic functions, like iron and zinc. Rather, heavy metals are contaminants in the body, interfering with enzymes and brain and organ function. They are typically difficult to get rid of. Some of these heavy metals are cadmium, lead and mercury, and one of the most pervasive, although not technically a heavy metal, is aluminum. It is able to cross the blood-brain barrier and has been implicated in autism and Alzheimer's disease, diseases of both young and old. Another modern pollutant is barium.

If not flushed from the body, metals can remain permanently enmeshed in the cells of the brain, bones, organs and soft tissues. They can take over sites that should be filled by other molecules and prevent proper function, and remain there until the tissues themselves are naturally replaced, which may take 15 years. According to a study published in Human Toxicology, these metals may not even show up on toxicity testing because they are not in the bloodstream, especially if infections are binding them. It may be impossible to flush them out unless the body is healthy, in which chelation is effective, over the course of months or years.

Barium sources include groundwater contamination, industrial pollution, smoking, fluorescent lights, electronics and, in recent years, from chemtrails, where it is heavily used. It can deplete potassium levels, with effects on the heart and cellular respiration, cause digestive dysfunction, high blood pressure, muscle twitching and weakness, and paralysis and possibly neurodegenerative diseases like multiple sclerosis. It can also lead to kidney damage or failure, respiratory failure and death. Barium was sprayed over war zones in the Middle Ease to sicken and weaken the enemy.

Mercury contamination in the body comes to us courtesy of dental amalgams, agricultural chemicals, polluted water, industrial processes including coal-burning plants, and fish that live in polluted waters. Mercury has also, finally, been acknowledged to be in vaccines and flu shots. The FDA has said that, because of complaints about the "theoretical" possibility of it being harmful, thimesoral has been almost entirely eliminated from vaccinations, but there is no way of knowing whether, assuming that is true, old stocks of vaccines are still being used. Mercury is also a component of compact fluorescent light bulbs (CFL's), and when they break they release mercury into the air. How many people know that if they break a CFL they are supposed to immediately evacuate the room, and open a window to air out the room for several hours? It's on an EPA web page, not on the package.

Aluminum is abundant in the earth, and may not be harmful if swallowed in dirt or clay. But we are overexposed to it in aluminum cookware, foil, frozen dinners and desserts, beverage cans and anti-perspirants. People living near aluminum plants suffer most, as they breathe it in. Aluminum is also found in chemtrails, another source of airborne pollution. Sadly, aluminum is the most common adjuvant in vaccines, even though it is a neurotoxin. It is especially dangerous to young children who, ironically, are the very persons who receive the most injections. Aluminum toxicity has not been sufficiently studied because, as the FDA admits, it was merely assumed that vaccines were not toxic. A 2011 study stated that it can have widespread and profound adverse health effects. It can cause bone weakness and disease, brain inflammation, neurological problems, muscle weakness and seizures, and is suspect in autism and Alzheimer's disease.

Lead remains a danger through old paint chips and painted window sashes (especially in older homes). Working in a plant that makes lead-containing items, or working with car batteries are sources of exposure. Some ceramic dishes may release lead. Fortunately, we no longer breathe leaded gas fumes, but lead is still a part of engine oil. Lead poisoning symptoms can include fatigue, constipation, decline in mental function, kidney disease, hypertension and miscarriage, among others.

Be Aware of Potential Exposure

Barium, aluminum, cadmium, strontium and other metals along with organic matter of all kinds are being sprayed in the atmosphere in chemtrails, for reasons never officially explained. Actually, the government denies their existence for the most part, but there are occasional slips, and the evidence of their existence and dire effects is abundant. Even if their only purpose were to reflect sunlight and slow global warming, as has been stated semi-officially, fine particles of aluminum and barium in our air is not a good thing. One early indicator of chemtrail effects is respiratory illnesses that don't respond to the usual treatments but may improve with metal cleansing. It's up to us to safeguard our own health.

Any heavy metal (or other non-biological molecule) will damage our health, whether we can identify specific symptoms or not. They clog our brains, cellular membranes, DNA and enzymes. Sometimes we simply operate at low energy and low brainpower and drag through life not realizing that we lack vitality. We must take heed to what we are eating, drinking and breathing and use beneficial foods and supplements to prevent metals from remaining in our bodies.

Glyphosate (and Other Chemicals)

Another very modern threat to our health is glyphosate. This is found in genetically engineered foods, which are themselves unnatural and unhealthy, and even in garden sprays. But glyphosate is a special threat for many reason. First, it kills beneficial bacteria in the gut, opening the door to all the consequences discussed in Chapters 5 and 7, including leaky gut, candida overgrowth and production of toxins by bad bacteria. Second, it facilitates the entry of aluminum into the body by helping it masquerade as calcium, so that it inserts itself into the places where calcium has metabolic functions, such as muscles and bones. A follow-on effect of that is calcification of the pineal gland. Third, preventing the normal metabolic functions of gut bacteria (not to say, killing them), deprives us of the indispensable vitamins and amino acids they produce for us. One notable effect is the depletion of the amino acid tryptophan, which is the sole precursor to melatonin, necessary for brain health. Fourth, it takes up residence itself in various tissues of the body and is hard to extricate, because it is a molecule not found in nature, so there are no means available to the body to deal with it. One place it gravitates to is bone tissue, where it replaces phosphorus, just as the aluminum it befriends takes the place of calcium. Fifth, researchers cite evidence that glyphosate may be the most significant cause of gluten intolerance and celiac disease, which are increasing dramatically in the U.S. Sixth, it is a potent chelator of vital trace minerals and destroyer of amino acids (tryptophan, methionine, tyrosine). Seventh, it interferes with the enzymes that detoxify drugs and synthesize cholesterol and sex hormones. Eighth, it cripples the immune system. This is not an exhaustive list; the point is to recognize the dangers of glyphosate and avoid it. There is apparently nothing that specifically detoxifies it, but it is to be hoped that the metal detoxification protocol outlined below will help. And Purification oil blend and Detoxyme are effective against most everything. But first, avoid GMO foods and other sources of glyphosate.

There are, obviously, innumerable other chemicals in our surroundings as we go through our daily lives. As with glyphosate, many are unnatural and toxic and difficult for our bodies to deal with. We live in an age where profit is more important to the few than the health of the many.

Chelators and Detoxifiers

A number of substances are effective against one or more heavy metals. If plentiful, magnesium protects against aluminum and other metals in brain cells, and helps prevent absorption of aluminum in the small intestine. Curcumin helps clear the amyloid plaques associated with Alzheimer's. Cilantro, chlorella and alpha-lipoic acid (ALA) can chelate mercury and lead. Malic acid (think raw apple cider vinegar) is good for aluminum, lead and strontium, while selenium is effective against mercury. Methionine, Vitamin C, garlic, MSM and calcium-sodium EDTA are additional metal chelators. Garlic and MSM are also sources of sulfur, which heavy metals prevent the brain from getting.

A Powerful, No-holds-barred metal cleanse

Here is a complete metal cleansing protocol. This cleanse picks up heavy metals, cleanses the liver, clears lymph, cleanses the kidney, and supports the spleen and adrenal glands. You want to have done colon and kidney cleanses before this metal cleanse, and preferably a Master Cleanse as well, to make sure the metals and toxins have a clear path to the exit.

This cleanse is a potent detoxifier. However, if you feel like you are detoxing too heavily, I urge you to use more JuvaCleanse and Detoxyme frequently throughout the day. Note that this cleanse is a 3-day repeating cycle.

DAY 1—Mobilizes metals.

- **First thing in morning upon arising:**
  Drink water
  Follow that with a tall glass of the following detoxifying lemonade drink:

  LEMONADE DRINK
  2 Tbl fresh squeezed lemon juice
  2 Tbl grade B maple syrup
  10 oz purified water
  1/8 tsp cayenne pepper

  And take these supplements:
  2 JuvaTone
  1 Comfortone
  2 Detoxzyme
  2 Essentialzyme-4
  2 L-Methionine 500 Mg
  1 Super B
  20 Drops of Juva Cleanse in a capsule (or if you choose to take it directly by mouth, i.e., by applying it to your inner cheek, you only need 3-4 drops, but do it 5 or 6 times a day.)

- **9 am**
  Do the spleen balance found in Ultimate Balance book. Use one of the oils listed in Ultimate Balance for spleen (i.e., Surrender, Release, Gratitude, Hope or Thieves)

  Drink 8 oz. fresh pineapple/grapefruit juice to clear spleen and lymph glands. **Add 2 drops of Grapefruit essential oil to the juice.**

- **10:45**
  Repeat spleen balance in Ultimate Balance

- **Lunch**
  Drink Powermeal or Pure Protein Complete, ideally in some sort of

fatty liquid, coconut milk, kefir, yogurt, etc. Add 4 drops of Frankincense, 4 drops of Copaiba, and 4 drops of Helichrysum, essential oils to the fatty liquid. The cream or fat in the liquid will mix with the oils and help them past the stomach acid into the small intestine.

Eat a salad with 1 tablespoon Juva Power mixed in.

Take 2 Essentialzyme-4

Drink 1 tablespoon ICP in juice and 2 oz NingXia Red (Drink NingXia Red throughout the day for blood sugar issues as needed.)

Also have some cilantro pesto. Eat it plain or mix in the salad or eat as a vegetable dip.

CILANTRO PESTO
   1 bunch cilantro, washed & dried
   3 cloves garlic
   1/2 c. olive oil
   1/2 tsp. salt
   1/2 tsp. pepper
   1/4 c. pine nuts (or another soft nut such as walnut or cashew)
   2 drops of Helichrysum essential oil
   3 drops of Coriander essential oil
   Mix ingredients in food processor until smooth.

- **1 pm**
  Do the small intestine energy balance in the Ultimate Balance book using one or more essential oils as listed in the book. (Hope, DiGize, Purification, Harmony, Peppermint)

- **2 pm**
  Drink Vital Life juice:

  VITAL LIFE JUICE
     3oz beet
     1oz celery
     1oz carrot
     1/3 oz Black Spanish radish (or Daigon radish or white radish)
     1/8th oz ginger root

1/3 oz red potato

4 oz cilantro

1 bud of garlic

2 drops of Coriander essential oil

All of the above in a blender. Please weigh the vegetables! If you use too much you can get very toxic.

Alternate the lemonade you made in the morning with this Vital Life juice every hour throughout the day as needed for detox or hunger. Eat Pesto also as needed for hunger.

- **2:45 pm**
Repeat small intestine balance.

    Have some kefir or yogurt with a drop or two of Melrose, Frankincense, Copaiba or Helichrysum mixed in it.

- **5 pm**
Do the kidney balance from Ultimate Balance with Juniper and Valor. Use K&B as needed.

    Eat a small dinner. Fish is best. Have more cilantro pesto and a salad with Power Meal. No wheat or gluten products

- **6:45 pm**
Repeat kidney balance.

Continue to alternate Vital Life juice and the lemonade juice as needed for hunger or detoxing.

- **9 pm and again at 10:345pm if you are awake**
Do the adrenal balance in Ultimate Balance, using one of the oils listed (Nutmeg, Endoflex, Hope, Surrender or Clove)

DAY 2—Detox day.

Eat fermented vegetables to bind metals and carry them out via the colon, use 1 Detoxyzme between meals, jump start Juva Cleanse as needed throughout the day. These will pull the metals you have mobilized out of the body. Eat normal meals, but no wheat or gluten products. Take Mineral Essence as directed on the bottle.

DAY 3—Rest day

Just eat normally again but no wheat or gluten products. (If needed, take the same detox supplements and oils as Day 2.) Take Mineral Essence as directed on the bottle.

DAY 4—A repeat of Day 1.

Begin to mobilize metals again and continue this cycle.

This is an amazing and very powerful liver cleanse and metal cleanse!

Regrettably, it isn't possible to explain the various balancing protocols in Ultimate Balance here, but basically you Vita-flex your feet, your organ alarm point, run the meridian and smell the oil. It is amazing how it tells the brain exactly what you want it to do. The book is available from Life Science Publishing.

If you feel toxic during the day, (achy, head-achy, achy in joints or bones, nauseous, etc) take a Detoxzyme pill and an L-Methionine pill and jump start Juva Cleanse until you feel better. Taking another Comfortone pill and a tablespoon of ICP in juice will also help. While not specifically mentioned in the above protocol, exercise is important to keep blood and lymph moving and body systems active so as to help get the metals going on their way.

Please note that when you are mobilizing heavy metals, the detox reaction can be quite intense. Blood purifiers such as red clover and yellow dock can help, as also do lemon enemas. The oil blends I generally recommend to help with clearing toxins from the blood are Juva Cleanse and Purification. In addition, using Methionine will assist in digesting metals quickly but it might also remove minerals. It is important to replace them on the off days.

How long should you stay on this cleanse? You will have to be the judge of that, base on how you feel. Everyone has different levels of metal contamination, so a hard and fast rule cannot be given. Hair and urine testing are an option, but the metals may not all be mobilized, yielding an inaccurate result. If you feel healthier, brighter and more energetic, you can probably stop this arduous cleanse and revert to a healthy lifestyle as a means to cleanse whatever is still in your body at a slower pace.

Stay Healthy

Given the many sources of metal contamination we are exposed to in our times, wisdom dictates that we pay close attention to what we take into our bodies or are exposed to. Avoid processed foods. It is worth the extra time to prepare food from healthful ingredients instead of buying things ready-made. Be sure to include plenty of fermented foods in your diet to carry toxins out of the digestive system and to boost beneficial gut bacteria. Both soluble (fermentable) and insoluble fiber as well as probiotics will also help maintain a healthy gut. Both macro and trace minerals are vital to keep our bodies functioning well and foreign metals out. Include in your normal diet the foods that chelate and flush metals mentioned earlier. Don't spray glyphosate on your vegetable garden. These are just a few steps we can take. More than ever, it's up to each individual and each family to watch out for our own health.

REFERENCES

Tomljenovic L, Shaw CA, Aluminum vaccine adjuvants: are they safe? Curr Med Chem. 2011;18(17):2630-7.

Tomljenovic L, Shaw CA, Mechanisms of aluminum adjuvant toxicity and autoimmunity in pediatric populations.Lupus. 2012 Feb;21(2):223-30. Doi: 10.1177/0961203311430221.

Domingo JL, Gómez M, Llobet JM, Corbella J.Comparative effects of several chelating agents on the toxicity, distribution and excretion of aluminium. Hum Toxicol. 1988 May;7(3):259-62.

Fiala M, et al Innate immunity and transcription of MGAT-III and Toll-like receptors in Alzheimer's disease patients are improved by bisdemethoxycurcumin. Proc Natl Acad Sci U S A. 2007 Jul 31;104(31):12849-54. Epub 2007 Jul 24.

Mike Adams, Cilantro helps detox heavy metals, http://www.naturalnews.com/027434_cilantro_natural_detox.html#ixzz2lETcHoWe

CHAPTER 11

Other Important Organs
(SUMMER)

When a person cleans the major eliminating organs of the body, namely, the colon, kidney and liver, 90 percent of his or her health problems seem to disappear. Generally the remaining organs also begin to clean themselves out because the way has been cleared for them to eliminate their waste products.

In our toxic society, it is a good practice to continually cleanse the body. Going through the cleansing cycle by season each year is an excellent idea. Reiterating what has been said in earlier chapters, clean the colon in the fall, the kidney in the winter and the liver in the spring. The following systems get their energies in the summer and should be cleansed and supported during that season.

Pancreas and Spleen

The pancreas and spleen share the same meridian in Chinese acupuncture even though one produces digestive enzymes and insulin and the other in in charge of the immune system of the body according to the ancient Chinese understanding. Interestingly enough, doing a liver cleanse assists both of these systems. The liver is the major sugar balancer of the body so cleansing it assists the pancreas in its role of insulin producer. Doing the Master Cleanse cleans receptor sites on the cells allowing insulin to enter; in other words, it clears up insulin resistance.

The pancreas responds well to Thieves oil. When it is sore or swollen, using Thieves in a warm compress over the area helps reduce inflammation.

Wolfberry products directly affect the pancreas: Sulferzyme and NingXia Red juice (both from Young Living) have yielded astonishing results with people who have had hypo- or hyperglycemia. I have personally used an ounce of NingXia Red juice every 15 minutes until my blood sugar stabilizes. (I used to use Berry Young juice until it was replaced by new and better NingXia Red.) I have also used NingXia Red to support the immune system when I have had the flu. This wonderful juice is amazingly high in antioxidants and also rich in vitamin C. More information about the pancreas and hypoglycemia is included in Chapter 12 on chronic fatigue.

An article in a 2005 journal states that the spleen combines the innate and adaptive immune systems, removing micro-organisms from the blood; it also serves as a reservoir for monocytes, which it deploys when the body receives a wound.

As mentioned above, cleaning the liver also assists the immune system. The reason for this is that the antibodies, which work to isolate and eliminate unfriendly bacteria and viruses, are primarily made from proteins. Therefore enhancing the liver's ability to metabolize proteins helps the body to make these protein-based antibodies.

The chart correlating organs and essential oils in Appendix B lists the oils that support the spleen and the pancreas.

Lymph

The best thing for maintaining lymphatic system function is to cleanse the major organs of elimination, because once the toxins have a pathway out of the body they will begin to leave the lymph glands or other tissues, enabling the lymph system to function more efficiently.

Many people do not realize how important the lymphatic system truly is. We never seem to think of it unless lymph nodes are swollen. Proteins and other cellular wastes which are too large to move through the capillaries to the veins are instead transported through the lymph system to the chest and then dumped into major blood vessels there. The lymph also carries with it any bacteria, viruses and fungi that have invaded body tissues, and passes them through lymph glands for detoxification along its way to the circulatory system and their eventual removal from the body.

If the lymphatic system were totally shut down we would die within 24 hours.

The lymph system needs to have a clear pathway for drainage. Sometimes it gets thick and full. This weakens the immune system and the body will begin to act like it has an illness as it tries to clear the sluggish lymph system on its own by raising a fever. Grapefruit essential oil and Ledum oil thin the lymph and help it to drain. A great recipe to use is a drop of Cypress, a drop of Orange oil and a drop of Grapefruit oil in a glass of water. Drink a glass at least 3 times a day. This is truly a remarkable cleanse for the lymph glands and will really help clear them out.

The Master Cleanse also helps to clear the lymph glands, but if you sense they are very swollen and full, try drinking this mixture along with the cleanse, or even alone if the need is urgent.

Not far from the gall bladder in the upper right quadrant of the abdomen sits the *cisterna chyli*. It is a very large lymph gland. The lymph from both legs, the lower part of the intestines and some thoracic sources all drain into it and from thence into the thoracic duct and on into the left subclavian vein. The cisterna chyli and thoracic duct can become quite full and may need to be manually drained using a vigorous massage. Many alternative health practitioners know how to do lymph drainage massages which are a great help to a clogged lymph system.

You can do a warm compress with the Cypress-Orange-Grapefruit oils combination or with Ledum oil over the cisterna chyli to help it drain.

Sometimes the cisterna chyli will become quite painful and mimic a gallbladder attack, since they are located so close to one another. However, pain from the cistern chyli usually does not refer to the right shoulder area the way gallbladder pain does. (Referred pain is felt in a place different than the pain's origin.) That said, if you think you are having a gallbladder attack, get a doctor's exam immediately. You don't want to self-diagnose yourself in this matter. Gallstones are a serious matter.

Using a body ionizer like the B.E.E.F.E.(Bio-electric Field Enhancement) will also help pull toxins from the lymph glands, and so will the hot bath with Epsom salts and Clove oil as mentioned in earlier chapters. Additionally, there are many acupressure points that can be stimulated to help drain this system. Rebounding on a mini tramp will always help the lymph system to move and is often recommended by doctors. Any strenuous exercise is a great help, as it causes both greater muscle activity and deeper breathing, both of which move the lymph.

Heart and Circulation System

The leading cause of death in the United States today is heart disease in one of its various forms. Much research point to diet and nutrition as the most powerful way to prevent or reverse heart disease. The heart needs calcium and other minerals to function optimally, and uses potassium and magnesium constantly. Many times when a patient comes in with heart palpitations or irregular heartbeat I find their problem stems from inadequate mineral intake in the diet. To avoid heart ailments, you have to be start by being conscious of the amount of these minerals you are getting in your diet or with supplementation, as well as trace minerals and essential amino acids.

Another little-known factor in heart health is fiber consumption. You recall from chapter 4 that Hippocrates said all disease begins in the colon. It appears that statement even applies to the heart: A pooled analysis of ten studies of dietary fiber intake in the U.S. and Europe found that each 10 grams per day increase in total dietary fiber intake was associated with a 14% decrease in the risk of myocardial infarction (heart attack), and a 24% decrease in deaths from coronary heart disease.

Many kinds of prescription drugs can damage heart tissue. Recent studies have shown that birth control pills may be a leading cause of heart disease in women today.

Smoking and alcohol consumption are two more major contributors to heart disease. It is vitally important to watch what you eat, how you rest, how you exercise, what you breathe and what you drink when it comes to heart health. Surprisingly, by-products of chlorination in our water supply have been identified as some of the worst causes of arteriosclerosis, heart attack and stroke. Stress, of course, is the number one cause of heart trouble. (See chapter 22.)

Cholesterol, on the other hand, is neither a cause nor an accurate indicator of circulatory problems. The hoopla about cholesterol in healthcare circles is a hoax, designed simply to make money. Our bodies make much more cholesterol than we get in our diet, because we need it for hormones, including sex hormones, for cell walls, nerves, bile salts and vitamin D – and to repair blood vessels. In my opinion the statin drugs prescribed to treat elevated cholesterol do much more harm than good. As far back as 2002 it was known that statins inhibit enzyme Co-Q10, which is necessary for muscle function (and the heart is a muscle). Supplementing with plain old magnesium, on the other hand, has been shown to lower LDL ("bad") cholesterol and raise HDL ("good") cholesterol, without the side effects of statins. Natural Calm from Natural Vitality is a good powdered magnesium supplement, available online, if you are concerned about cholesterol. It would be much safer than statin drugs, and our bodies probably are not getting all the magnesium they require anyway.

We need to understand that natural fats and oils are good for us. To prevent plaqueing (hardening) of the arteries, also known as atherosclerosis, the best idea is probably a diet rich in the fat-soluble vitamins A, D and K, and essential fatty acids. Animal fats are important; these help prevent inflammation, which is behind plaqueing, but polyunsaturated vegetable oils are problematic. Fluoride is known to promote inflammation,so obviously fluoridated toothpaste cannot be good for our arteries. The chlorine in our municipal water supplies reacts with organic matter (leaves, twigs) and agricultural runoff to create trihalomethanes, which Dr. Joseph M. Price warns are the prime causes of arteriosclerosis.

OmegaGize from Young Living is excellent to support cardiovascular health. The bottle recommends 4 capsules a day, but if you are symptomatic, take up to 8 a day. By symptomatic I mean you may suffer from poor memory, foggy thinking,hormonal disruption, depression, dry hair and skin, or dry colon. These obviously are not cardiovascular issues, but if you have these things going on, you most likely are running low on essential fatty acids, and you also need them for cardiovascular health – sort of like a canary in a coal mine.

Salt is falsely accused of being an enemy of cardiovascular health. Although everyone "knows" that we need to restrict salt intake for our heart's sake, it just isn't true. The FDA will persist in saying otherwise, but very careful research, done without jumping to conclusions, does not show sodium chloride (salt) to be detrimental to heart health, but rather that restricted sodium intake is a health risk. (The chloride part of salt also provides a necessary part of stomach acid, HCl.) As a matter of note, when Americans used to average twice as much salt consumption as we do now, partly through eating meats preserved in salt, they had much less of heart disease. There really is no connection between salt and cardiovascular disease, although, as in so many other health topics, it can be very difficult for most people to parse out where the pseudo-scientific errors lie.

Clogged arteries and veins are a serious problem that restricts bloodflow to the heart, depriving it of essential oxygen This is the primary cause of heart attacks. Medical doctors typically prescribe synthetic blood thinners for people with circulatory problems to keep clots from blocking a cardiac artery or vein. Better, natural alternatives as blood thinners, if you need them, include aged garlic and vitamin E. Cayenne pepper and both Clove and Cistus essential oils are other natural substances that will thin the blood.

CardiaCare and HRT are two additional Young Living products that support the heart. Remember also to drink plenty of water.

I had a patient who, under the supervision of her medical doctor, was able to get off all her medications, which included diuretics, blood pressure medications and heart medications after she did a colon cleanse, a liver cleanse and the Master Cleanse. She did all these cleanses while still on her medications, and began using essential oils, CardiaCare and HRT before her doctor started cutting back her medications. She is now off medications and is maintaining her heart health very well by using the above products. I do not recommend you attempt something so drastic on your own without the help of knowledgeable, trained physicians who know how to advise you on the cleanses and also how to ease you off your medications at the right time, if that is advisable for you. It is dangerous to go off medications suddenly. Many have to be cut back gradually to prevent serious withdrawal effects.

One of the reasons for clogged veins and arteries is that the liver is not handling fats and/or proteins well. As a result, the excess fats and proteins are more likely to oxidize in the body, creating plaque, thickening the blood and raising the potential for blood clots. Further, if the body isn't getting the proper nutrients the artery and vein walls can become weak and stretch, creating aneurysms and varicose veins.

One excellent way to help clean up the circulatory system is to cleanse the liver, take enzymes and drink NingXia Red juice. NingXia Red juice helps balance the blood sugar and other blood chemistries. For years, I have personally battled lupus. During one lupus flare, I was having problems with dizziness and blackouts. A darkfield microscopy analysis of my blood showed it to be extremely thick, with large amounts of plaque, undigested proteins and fats and incomplete sugar digestion. The red blood cells were being destroyed by free radicals. A doctor wanted me to do chelation therapy immediately to clear out the blood and prevent a heart attack or stroke. I chose instead to go home and drink a quarter cup of Berry Young Juice hourly. (Berry Young was an older Young Living product; now there's NingXia Red juice, which is even better.) Within three days, the dizziness and blackout spells were over. My blood looked healthy again. I then did a liver cleanse and took enzyme supplements to help heal my liver and increase its functionality.

To help shrink varicose veins, it is important to first do a colon and liver cleanse (I can't seem to say this enough). A dirty, clogged colon leads to constipation, which puts a lot of pressure on the veins and arteries of the legs so the blood doesn't flow properly; this also leads to weak veins that can't move the blood back up to the heart properly. A good diet with plenty of fiber is essential for good colon health, which is a must for vein health. Following the cleanses, I recommend that my patients take flax seed oil, vitamin E, calcium, potassium, phosphorous and vitamin C to strengthen the veins. It is also important to ensure that your spine and pelvis are in good alignment so that the nerve supply to the lower extremities is functioning optimally and is not restricted.

Enzyme supplements, especially Essentialzyme or Essentialzymes-4 taken between meals will help clear out the plaque that is lining the walls of the arteries and veins.

I personally think everyone would be well-advised to take ICP for their entire lives just to make sure they are getting plenty of fiber. Fiber is extremely important, as we saw in Chapter 4. an analysis of ten studies revealed that each additional 10 grams per day of fiber resulted in a 24 percent decrease in deaths from coronary disease. I try to take 2 Tbs of a green food drink mixed with 1 Tbs of ICP and 1 Tbs of ground flax meal twice a day. It seems to keep the acids out of my joints and gives me plenty of fiber and Omega-3 fatty acids. This drink keeps rheumatoid and lupus arthritis from swelling up in my joints so I don't wake up stiff and in pain in the mornings. It also seems to keep my veins from swelling from lupus during the day.

As a lupus sufferer, I find that Australian Blue and Idaho Balsam Fir help decrease vein swelling. Another thing that helps decrease vein swelling is NingXia Red juice. Many times vasculitis is caused by the excessive release of histamines. NingXia Red juice is, among its other virtues, an excellent antihistamine and helps control that part of the immune system.

Clots can be dissolved using warm compresses of Cistus or Helichrysum oils. I have also had great results dissolving clots with Tei Fu oil from Nature's Sunshine, applied topically.

Stomach and small intestine

In Chapter 4 we discussed the digestive system and its functions. Generally speaking a good colon cleanse like the one outlined in Chapter 4 and the Master Cleanse (Chapter 7) clean the stomach and the small intestine at the same time as the colon, and if there are parasites in the small intestine the parasite cleanse (Chapter 4) will take care of them. Therefore all we really need to discuss about the stomach and small intestine here is how to support them.

As stated in chapter 4, the stomach produces hydrochloric acid (HCl) to aid in protein digestion. This acid also serves another very important purpose, that of helping destroy bacteria, viruses, parasites and fungi that are swallowed with our food. If a person is having trouble with indigestion (particularly with regard to proteins), which sometimes happens as we approach middle age, it is most often due to <u>low</u> acidity of the stomach, NOT excess acid as is so commonly suggested in advertising. One study showed that production of HCl averages 180 ml/hour in teenagers, but drops to only 50ml/hour by the time we reach our 60's. As a result of low stomach acidity, food will sit longer in the stomach and begin to putrify or ferment, causing gas and pain and – surprise! – "acid reflux." So don't take drugs or antacids to treat excess acid; that's the opposite of what you need.

Although the stomach needs acid to digest protein and as a first line of defense against micro-organisms, as we age, leaving the main growth phase of life and typically engaging in less vigorous activity, our bodies are genetically programmed to expect less protein, so our stomachs produce less acid. Most people, according to the simplest calculations, actually require 2 ounces or less of protein per day (pregnant or lactating women need 3 ounces). That's the equivalent of only half a quarter-pounder. Most of us easily get enough protein in our diets. However, many people eat more than is biologically necessary or expected, and the amount of stomach acid produced doesn't keep up. Taking a supplement called Betaine HCl (found at most health food stores) will usually take care of the "heartburn" problem. Often it isn't necessary to take it all the time; the body seems to get restarted on its own once given some encouragement and an occasional boost. If HCL alone doesn't solve the problem, adding a protease enzyme (see Appendix C) will assist the stomach and small intestine to digest protein.

Prescription and over-the-counter drugs for "acid indigestion" and "heartburn" are not only a misguided approach, but pharmaceuticals typically only mask symptoms anyway, and they introduce side-effects, such as impaired thinking created by the anti-cholinergic action of many drugs, including antacids (acetylcholine is the main neurotransmitter used in the brain and nervous system). And over-the-counter antacids create a reduction in stomach acid that impairs protein digestion and allows dangerous micro-organisms to pass into the small intestine.

The chemical compounds in these drugs also facilitate yeast growth; candida is normally kept in check by acidity, but it can colonize the stomach under conditions of low acidity, following which the consumption of sugary foods will cause foaming as the yeast feeds on it, which creates pressure on the cardiac sphincter: more acid reflux. Candida can go so far as to take up residence on the esophageal valve thank to low stomach acidity and prevent its proper closing. Then you get even more reflux.

As a matter of fact, consumption of aspirin, alcohol, cigarettes and coffee is frequently to blame for acid stomach symptoms and ought to be addressed first. The problem certainly doesn't stem from a lack of drugs in the system; just the opposite. And the American Medical Association has warned that people using common drugs that suppress stomach acid have an increased risk of fractures, serious intestinal infections and pneumonia.

Another unrecognized factor is that acid reflux and other such digestive problems are often merely the natural result of over-eating, especially consistent over-eating that leads to big bellies that push the cardiac valve at the top of the stomach up through the diaphragm. Straining at the toilet can cause the same thing. This condition, called hiatal hernia, allows stomach acid to be forced into the esophagus, which eventually can lead to health problems much more severe than the discomfort we experience from heartburn. Hiatal hernia can often be treated non-surgically by a chiropractor who has been taught about this condition. Nighttime incidents of acid reflux can be greatly reduced by refraining from eating after dinner. Meanwhile, in cases of, for example, heartburn from spicy foods, sniffing Wintergreen or Peppermint oil should be your first option, and taking one drop of Peppermint oil in a cup of water should relieve a more serious bout.

The small intestine, liver and pancreas are responsible for sending enzymes to the upper part of the small intestine, the duodenum, to continue the digestive processes for proteins as well as to digest fats and carbohydrates. Enzymes are the primary factor in digestion, and a person who lacks enzymes can be literally starving and suffering all manner of nutritional-deficiency diseases even though eating a lot of food. If you are experiencing bloating or stomachaches after eating and it doesn't stem from an anatomical/physiological problem, you should probably take enzymes with your meals. Processed foods are bereft of enzymes, making their digestion more difficult, depending as it does entirely on your own self-produced enzymes, or on supplements. See appendix C for a list of Young Living enzymes and their purposes.

Small Intestine Bacterial Overgrowth

Insufficient acidity of the stomach is a contributing factor to small intestine bacterial overgrowth (SIBO), a condition in which microorganisms (mainly yeast) that should exist only in small numbers in the small intestine have multiplied beyond the norm. The colon cleanse and Master Cleanse protocols should take care of this but if the condition comes up as a problem that you want to deal with specifically, it can be easily done.

The primary symptoms of SIBO are similar to IBS symptoms, including:

- Abdominal bloating
- Belching
- Gas
- Abdominal pain

- Cramping
- Constipation
- Diarrhea

Leaky gut symptoms are also a big sign of SIBO. These can range from food sensitivities to headaches, fatigue, skin issues, mood issues, asthma, and joint pain.

Even though the best way to use essential oils against yeast in the large intestine or colon, where most of it is, is through rectal injections; in the small intestine (SIBO), it is best handled by mouth. The same oils used for the large intestine or colon are useful for the small intestine. One such oil is Melrose, which you can take in capsules (25 drops in a capsule 3 times a day), or 15 drops in one Tbs of coconut oil, flax seed oil, cream or another fatty oil, which will help get the oil past the stomach and into the small intestine where they will then spread through the system and handle the yeast problems there. Coconut oil is probably the best option, because it has anti-fungal properties of its own. You can add this to a smoothie if you prefer. Cedarwood and Pachouli can be used this way too.

Hot oils such as Thyme and Lemongrass need to be more dilute, only 7 drops to a Tbs. of coconut oil, before taking them internally, either rectally or in a smoothie or just swallowed down. Using these oils emulsified in a fatty oil such as cream, flax seed oil, coconut oil etc, and mixing them into a smoothie, will assist them in bypassing the stomach and go directly into the small intestine.

With any of these oils, continue the protocol until symptoms disappear. Many times that includes losing inches of bloat off the abdomen.

Stress has been found to be a major factor in SIBO, just as it is in irritable bowel syndrome (IBS). Cortisol, released by the adrenal glands in response to stress, slows activity in the upper bowel and over-stimulates the colon.

There are many "natural" ways of dealing with stress, including, as we discussed in Chapter 5, having healthy gut flora. Please see Chapter 22 for further ideas about dealing with stress. Please don't take anti-depressants.

Gall Bladder

The gall bladder is closely associated with the liver, and cleansing the liver also works to cleanse the gall bladder. Technically, the gall bladder would be cleansed, in conjunction with the liver, during the spring, and usually does not require any targeted cleansing protocol per se, but I slipped it into this chapter with the summer systems to add some important information that is specific to it.

There are techniques for draining and cleansing the gall bladder that go beyond the directions for a general liver cleanse. It is probably a wise approach to gall bladder health to simply take Ledum oil periodically as it helps to drain the gall bladder. Juva Flex is an oil blend that also helps to thin bile and drain the gall bladder. You can either take it internally or use it as a compress over the gall bladder area. Since some people have complained of having gall bladder pain after doing the Master Cleanse, I suggest using Ledum oil and Juva Flex while on the cleanse to help keep the gall bladder clear. However, these supposed gall bladder attacks may actually have been a filled cisterna chyli—see the section on lymph earlier in this chapter.

There is another gall bladder flush that calls for drinking apple juice for several days followed by Epsom salts and an olive oil/grapefruit drink. Though I know several people who have successfully used this flush to clean out gallstones, some doctors recommend against it because it has the potential to force out large stones that may get stuck in the gall bladder's bile duct, leading to emergency gall bladder surgery. Another concern with this flush is the potential for the magnesium in the Epsom salts to depress the heart rate too much, again creating a need for emergency intervention. Before using this type of flush it would be wise to drain the lymph system as discussed later in the chapter, and also to take Ledum and Juva Cleanse oils for a few days before and again during the flush to help keep the bile and lymph thin and free-flowing. I find that by keeping the bowel and the liver cleansed the bile has an easy outlet and has fewer tendencies to stagnate and create stones, thus eliminating the need to do a specific gallbladder flush. However, if you do want to do a gallbladder flush and are sure you can deal with any problems that may arise, the instructions are given in Appendix D at the back of the book. I have included it for the sake of completeness, but I don't generally recommend it.

Case history

Elizabeth came to my office after a severe traffic accident. While treating her, I taught her about natural healing. She told me about her health problems. She had been on Erythromycin for 12 years for a pain in her chest and felt that if she went off the antibiotic the pain in her chest would come back she had no idea what it was. She was on nin different medications for congestive heart failure which included heart medication, blood pressure medication and a diuretic.

I called a D.O. Friend of mine who also works with Young Living Oils and gave him the list of medications, asking him if he thought it was possible to use cleanses while on these drugs. He stated that is was indeed possible and encouraged me to put her on a colon cleanse and the Master Cleanse immediately. She agreed to go on the cleanses. I also put her on Cardia Care and HRT. I asked her to go to her medical doctor and talk to him about taking her off the antibiotic and the diuretic. She did so and he agreed to let her go off those two drugs. While on the Master Cleanse she began to lose a lot of water. In fact, she lost so much water that her swollen ankles came down to normal size again - something that she had not experienced while on the diuretic, interestingly enough. She never had another problem with the pain in her chest and eventually was able to go off all nine medications that she had been on. I had her do a yeast cleanse following closely after the other cleanses because she had been on so many medications for so long.

She loved the Master Cleanse so much that she would repeat it for one week out of every month just to make sure that her body didn't accumulate water or toxins.

REFERENCES

Worsley, J.R., Traditional Chinese Acupuncture Vol. 1: Meridians and Points (2nd ed.), Element Books Ltd, Rockport MA 1993

Guyton, Arthur C. Textbook of Medical Physiology. W.B. Saunders Company. Philadelphia PA. 1991

Tabers Cyclopedic Medical Dictionary, Clayton L. Thomas MD, MPH ed., F.A. Davis Co. Philadelphia PA 1993

National Center for Health Statistics, Centers for Disease Control http://www.cdc.gov/nchs/fastats/lcod.htm

Boyles, Salynn, The Pill Linked to Heart Disease Protein, http://www.webmd.com/content/article/63/72071.htm

Champagne ET. Low gastric hydrochloric acid secretion and mineral bioavailability. Adv Exp Med Biol. 1989;249:173-84.

Betaine (HCl), Anti-Aging Library, American Academy of Anti-Aging Medicine, http://www.worldhealth.net/p/aadr-betaine-hcl.html

Essential Oils Desk Reference 3rd ed., Essential Science Publishing, USA 2004

Mönnikes H1, Tebbe JJ, et al. Role of stress in functional gastrointestinal disorders. Evidence for stress-induced alterations in gastrointestinal motility and sensitivity. 2001;19Dig Dis.(3):201-11.

Tachee Y, Kiank C, Stengel A. A Role for Corticotropin-releasing Factor in Functional Gastrointestinal Disorders. Curr Gastroenterol Rep. Aug 2009; 11(4): 270–277.

Collins SM, Bercik P. The relationship between intestinal microbiota and the central nervous system in normal gastrointestinal function and disease. Gastroenterology. 2009 May;136(6):2003-14. doi: 10.1053/j.gastro.2009.01.075. Epub 2009 May 7.

Health Effect of Chlorine in Drinking Water http://www.pure-earth.com/chlorine.html

Mebius, RE; Kraal, G (2005). "Structure and function of the spleen". Nature reviews. Immunology 5 (8): 606–16

Swirski, FK; Nahrendorf, M; et al. (2009). "Identification of splenic reservoir monocytes and their deployment to inflammatory sites". Science 325 (5940): 612–6.

CHAPTER 12

Colon and Lungs…Again
(FALL)

We have come full circle now with the seasons of the year. We started in the fall with the colon. In the winter we cleaned the kidney followed by the the yeast/parasite cleanse and the Master Cleanse. In the spring we took care of the liver and gall bladder. In the summer we cleared out the lymph system and supported the heart and other organs.

While I have left the lungs and the skin until the second fall, after all the other organs, they will almost always noticeably clear up when you clean the colon. It is amazing how much a colon cleanse assists the lungs. Many times when there is a lung problem we clean the colon first. If you want to affect the lungs in any way, it is powerful to use the colon as an entry point by giving enemas or oils that assist the lungs by means of cold water injections, through the rectum into the colon. Even though I am only now getting around to mentioning the lungs and skin here, it is important to know that you can clean them and support them at the same time that you clean the colon.

Lungs

The lungs are an extremely delicate tissue. They can be damaged easily by cigarette smoke or other pollutants and by breathing in dust or fine particles. It has been said that once damaged, lung tissue doesn't repair itself. I still hold to the belief that if given the proper nutrients and therapies the body will heal itself.

Recently the effectiveness of citrus oils in stopping asthma attacks was in the news. Many of my patients whose children had asthma started using Citrus Fresh oil just around the child's pillow at nighttime and much to their delight, the asthma attacks dwindled. Some have been so bold as to mix Citrus Fresh with water and use it in the child's nebulizer instead of Albuterol. It worked there too.

Asthma like other allergies, is thought to be related to liver and adrenal insufficiency. It is alleviated to a great extent by supporting the adrenals with Nutmeg essential oil, Super B and Mineral Essence.

On a personal note, it was a bout with pneumonia that started my natural healing experience. I had never used herbs but was interested in them, so I signed up for a natural healing class and ordered some books. The same day that my books on how to use herbs arrived in the mail, my 2-year-old son was diagnosed with pneumonia. I went home from the medical doctor's office with the prescription drug and met the mailman delivering my herbal medicine books. I stood there with the books in one hand and the antibiotic in the other. Here indeed was a moment of decision.

The herbal treatment the books recommended for pneumonia was long, hard to do, and involved something called "The Cold Sheet Treatment" (See Appendix E). Interestingly enough, it starts by cleaning out the patient's colon! We first gave peppermint enemas to clear out the old debris and to relax the colon so it wouldn't spasm for the next enema. The next enema was a garlic/lemon juice/cold water injection to draw mucus out of the body, and it certainly did that. Strings of mucus came out of his colon, cups and cups of it. Then we bathed my little patient in warm water with cayenne pepper, dry mustard and ginger to help his body to raise its temperature. The reason for this was that a fever helps the body increase its white blood count and is also thought to help fight infection directly.

We gave him feverfew or peppermint tea to drink to make him break out in a sweat. As soon as he did we wrapped him naked in a cold wet sheet, and then covered him with large warm woolen blankets to keep the fever wet and working. Next we smeared Vaseline and chopped garlic on his feet as an antibiotic and wrapped his feet in rags. (Garlic is a powerful antibiotic; the Vaseline was just there to keep the garlic stuck to the feet.)

Imagine me, as a mother, brand-new to natural health care, giving my 2-year-old baby boy this treatment instead of antibiotics and lying awake all night thinking that I had potentially made an enormous mistake! You can imagine my delight, both as a caregiver and as a mother, when in the morning, the child awoke stinking like burnt hair or rubber and his diaper was full of thick brown mucus—but his lungs were as clear as a bell. The infection had left the body and the child was well!

As mentioned above the lungs have a direct relationship with the colon in the Law of the 5 Elements: They are the yin and yang, respectively, of the Metal element. Clean the colon and you clean the lungs! If the colon is full of mucus the lungs can't get rid of their mucus.

Of course the lungs create a certain amount of mucus normally to pick up the toxins and dust that we breathe in through the nose, most of which is expelled through the nose's mucous membrane. The sinuses and nose keep the air warm and moist so it won't dry out the lung tissue. An excess of processed dairy products fills the intestinal tract with mucus and causes an overproduction of mucus throughout the body. I have observed that people who stop drinking cow's milk also stop having bronchitis, asthma, pneumonia, ear infections, sinusitis and hyperactivity.

We have had surprising success with an essential oil mixture to get rid of congestion in the lungs. We make a blend of 3 drops of Marjoram essential oil, 3 drops of Juva Cleanse oil blend and 1 drop of Lavender essential oil. (Yes, it's true that a liver cleanser (Juva Cleanse) is part of this expectorant. And it really works!) I have my patients smell the oil, put a drop in the lining of the cheek several times a day, and make a warm compress to put over the chest. Results are almost immediate.

Whenever I feel that tickle in the back of my throat that tells me a cold or cough is trying to start, I immediately take one capsule full of Oregano oil, diluted 50-50 in vegetable oil, and go to bed. Usually by morning the chest is clear and the cold or virus is gone. Oregano oil is fabulous for the lungs. I think it should be used with all lung ailments.

We have also used a blend of Oregano or Thyme with Peppermint and Melrose, RC or Raven in a sinus facial steamer to get the oils inhaled deeply into the sinuses and lungs. People have worried that the heat from the steam might destroy some of the active ingredients in the oils, and it may to some extent, but it certainly still has some healing value left since it works wonderfully!

Sinusitis is easy to treat by putting a drop of RC or Eucalyptus oil on the gums under the upper lip every minute for 10 minutes then every 10 minutes for an hour, then every hour for the rest of the day. The sinuses usually begin to clear up during the first 20 minutes.

An old-fashioned remedy is to make a saline solution of ½ tsp salt to one cup of warm water, then drop 2-3 drops of this solution in the nose as needed through out the day. Imagine my surprise when I learned that our local children's hospital uses this saline solution on the children instead of commercial decongestants. When I asked the nurses about it, they said that both decongestant sprays and children's liquid cough formulas have a rebound effect that does not occur with the saline solution. A rebound effect is when the initial symptoms go away but then they return again in greater force once treatment stops.

The Skin

The skin, as the largest organ of the body, has several important functions, the most obvious one being that of a protective surface covering over the body. It also has been called the second kidney or the second lung. If observed carefully, it can give us clues as to what is happening elsewhere in the body.

Skin eruptions have been attributed to both the liver and the colon. According to the Five Elements law, the skin is under the management of the colon. Skin rashes that are not viral in origin are usually the result of a dirty colon. The skin will erupt with yeast or mold patches or fungi if the colon needs to be cleaned. Eczema and psoriasis have been attributed to a clogged colon too. After a thorough cleaning of the colon many patients have been completely cleared of these problems.

Brown or red spots appear on the skin if the liver needs cleansing. The skin often becomes itchy if the colon, liver and kidney are not clearing their toxins as they should. In other words, if the body cannot eliminate its wastes through proper channels it will send them out through the skin. If that is not possible, it will store them in body tissues, especially fatty tissues, either around organs or under the skin.

The skin produces mast cells, which are the first white blood cells to be activated in the immune system response. The mast cells release histamines to start the healing process and to signal other white blood cells to come to the area. When the digestive system is clogged and not digesting its proteins properly, as mentioned in an earlier chapter, the body can break out in an allergic attack if confronted with a foreign protein. Often this manifests in hives on the skin. This problem can be completely taken care of by cleansing the digestive system, but for symptomatic relief, Lavender essential oil, RC blend and Australian Blue blend are good contact antihistamines to help control hives.

Ningxia Red is so full of vitamin C that it is an excellent antihistamine. Take ¼ cup every hour until the reaction is gone.

My teenage son had horrible allergies but wasn't willing to do a liver or colon cleanse to get rid of them. I was away from home when he called me to tell this story: He had gone into a barn full of moldy hay and while there got stung by a bee. He immediately swelled up. He had an asthma attack. His nose started running. He broke out in hives and on top of all that he had huge three-inch welts all over his body. He had difficulty breathing and was just about unable to speak. Fortunately he was standing by my buffet that had all my oils on top of it. I told him to grab the RC and Peppermint oils and start breathing them. I started for home and stayed on the phone with him until I could hear that his breathing was better and his asthma had relaxed. Then I told him to rub Lavender all over himself and to start taking the Lavender and some Juva Cleanse by mouth, each a drop at a time for a minute then every ten minutes until I got home. When I got there fifteen minutes later, his breathing was much better but he was still covered in welts and hives. I ran bath water and put Lavender water and Lavender oil and him in it. I gave him 5 JuvaTone capsules and started him on Ningxia Red, 2 Tablespoons every 15 minutes. Within about 15 minutes of taking the first dose of Ningxia Red, the hives and welts began to disappear. This dramatic experience made him a believer in the oils— and he went on a colon and liver cleanse the next day.

The skin is a major temperature regulator of the body, but if it can't breathe because of blocked pores the body will have a difficult time in extreme weather. Skin lotions, suntan lotions, moisturizing soaps and other products clog the skin. As previously stated, if the colon, liver or kidneys are unable to eliminate their toxins through their regular routes, the body will attempt to get rid of the toxins through the skin, and if the skin is smothered in lotions and so forth, the result will be clogged pores skin infections, acne and blemishes.

Additionally, it is vital that the skin be able to receive sunlight in order to make vitamin D, which is essential for absorption of calcium in the bones. Some studies have shown that incorporating cooked tomato products in the diet has some effect on protecting from ultra-violet radiation as do <u>natural</u> beta-carotenes, vitamin E and vitamin C, when eaten consistently. That doesn't mean you can swallow some spaghetti and vitamins for breakfast and go spend the day in the sun! But a healthy diet containing plenty of vitamins and anti-oxidants and moderate sun exposure is a much healthier choice than processed factory foods and sunscreen.

Young Living Essential Oils has a line of products call Age Refining Technology (A.R.T.) formulated to recover the skin from damage caused by exposure to the sun and from aging processes. These products contain essential oils that replenish DNA and liposomes to carry active ingredients into the lower layers of the skin.

To clear the skin it must be dry-brushed with a loofah every day in the direction of the heart. Then I like to use a good soap like Thieves soap or Miracle II soap to cleanse the skin while it is still dry. Let the soap work for a few minutes, then get in a warm-to-hot shower to rinse off. Follow that with a cold spray to stimulate and invigorate the pores of the skin. Give the skin a shallow massage all over to loosen it and allow it to release its toxins.

Soaking in Epsom salts and a few drops of Clove oil will help draw toxins out of the skin. One patient reported that after laying 15 minutes in a tub full of water and 10 drops of Clove oil, her skin suddenly became itchy all over and a dark, sticky ooze started coming out of the pores. Give the skin a vigorous rub with one of the good glycerin bars made by Young Living Essential Oils or with Miracle II soap to rid the skin of this buildup of toxins.

Strenuous exercise is good for overall health and good for the skin as it helps it to sweat and rid itself of unwanted toxins. Steam baths, saunas, sweat lodges and so forth are very effective.

Don't forget to replace your electrolytes with Mineral Essence if you sweat a lot. If you don't sweat during exercise or on a hot day, your skin is clogged and unable to get rid of toxins, so you need to do a skin cleanse. There are also herbal wraps that help pull toxins from the skin. The Master Cleanse is an excellent skin cleanser.

I personally went through an accidental skin cleanse several years ago, and I was astonished at the toxins that came out of my skin. It occurred as an unexpected by-product of using an herbal product called BF&C (by Dr. Christopher) for a broken leg.

I learned a lot about what can be stored just under the skin from that cleanse. I had had a rash for years prior to that time, right along the band of my bra. It was red and very itchy. During this cleanse, I broke out in bands of red and yellow and blue across my abdomen. The red strip was right under my bra.

I realized that this was where my body stored food colorings. I had for several years taken a lot of little red pills for sinus problems, and that is where the red dye was apparently stored. Not being a natural substance, my body could not metabolize those pills and had to store the dyes in them subdermally, in the fat layer just under the skin.

But that was only the beginning. I started noticing tiny wood slivers and glass pieces coming out of my hands and feet, things the body had not been able to get rid of and had built protection around. The most amazing thing was that I started to smell like vapor rub and its greasy feeling manifested on my chest and back. I washed it off and more came out. Even makeup started coming out of the pores on my face. My husband complained that I was wearing my makeup too thick when I hadn't even put any on. I washed it off just to have it reappear! The black circles under my eyes turned out to be mascara streaks (from years of wearing makeup to bed).

I also began to burp up antacid flavorings and I even recognized the flavor of a medication that I used to take in my teenage years for stomach upset. That would have been twenty years earlier. The list goes on. It seemed that every medication that I had taken either came out through the skin or up through the stomach.

The next thing that happened was I started to get symptoms of infections I had had again (breast infections, lung infections, sinus infections, kidney infections). This time instead of running for an antibiotic, however, I used herbs, including garlic and other microbe-killing herbs to combat the infections. I decided that instead of using drugs to suppress the symptoms, I would do it right this time and completely heal the problem. These very unusual symptoms lasted almost two weeks..

What I learned from all of this was that toxins (including medications, makeup and other unnatural substances) can and do get stored in the tissues of the body. They store in the fat cells in places close to where they are being used or accumulate together in "storage units" like the food-coloring bands on my abdomen. They store because, being unnatural, the body has no way to deal with them.

I have been told by others who have used herbal wraps, the Master Cleanse or the cold sheet treatment that they have experienced similar symptoms as the skin began to cleanse itself.

REFERENCES

Connelly, Dianne M. PhD, Traditional Acupuncture: The Law of Five Elements. Traditional Acupucture Institute Columbia, MD. 1994

Essential Oils Desk Reference 3rd ed., Essential Science Publishing, USA 2004

Guyton, Arthur C. Textbook of Medical Physiology. W.B. Saunders Company. Philadelphia PA. 1991

Citrus Oil for Asthma?, American Technion Society CONNECTIONS Electronic Newsletter December 29, 2004 http://www.ats.org/newsletters.php?id=70

Skin, American Medical Association Professional Resources Atlas of the Body, http://www.ama-assn.org/ama/pub/category/7176.html

Monte Kline, Ph.D., Skin Problems, Pacific Health Center Better Health Update 45, http://www.pacifichealthcenter.com/updates/45.asp

Stahl, W. et al, Dietary tomato paste protects against ultraviolet light-induced erythema in humans, J Nutr. 2001 May;131(5):1449-51

CHAPTER 13

Don't Forget Me!
(Other Body Systems That May Need Attention)

The systems of the body discussed in this chapter generally clear up during the Master Cleanse. I have included them here to complete the picture of cleansing the entire body. Consult the afterword on any particular season of the year in which to clean them, otherwise use this chapter as a general guideline on how to support these systems.

Muscles

I have noticed in my practice that there are six principal reasons for muscle soreness.

1. Stress
2. Lack of calcium and/or magnesium
3. Lack of exercise
4. Overexertion
5. Toxic buildup
6. Spine out of alignment

All of these problems are relatively easy to fix. Decrease stress through relaxation techniques. Go to a massage therapist. Eat a good diet. Take good calcium and magnesium supplements. Exercise regularly. Properly stretch your muscles out before and after any vigorous exercise (including any heavy, strenuous work). Utilize the cleansing techniques discussed in this book. See your chiropractor.

Raindrop technique is a very effective muscle relaxer and helps release toxins from the muscles. I also love to put Clove oil, Aroma Seiz blend, Peace and Calming blend or Marjoram in the bathtub to relax muscles. Regenolone cream is excellent for sprains and strains.

As a chiropractor, I have observed that if someone is not responding to chiropractic care and continues to have tight muscles after several treatments, that patient needs a colon cleanse to help clean out toxins in the muscles.

For example, one of my patients was stopped at a red light and was rear-ended. The other driver was probably only going 10-15 miles an hour. But my patient suffered a tremendous whiplash that affected her whole spine. (Low-speed collisions often cause a surprising amount of trauma to the spine.) Her back was extremely tight and would not respond to chiropractic treatment even combined with Raindrop technique. She was not able to go to work because of the intense pain in her low and mid back. She had horrible breath, so bad that I felt like her entire "sewer system" was backed up. Upon questioning her I discovered that she was only having one bowel movement a week and had been like that for years. I kept suggesting to her that she do a colon cleanse but since she had never done one before she was not open to the idea. The automobile insurance company finally decided to settle the account and give her a disability rating since she couldn't seem to heal from the accident. After she started having to pay for her own care she became more interested in what she could do to help herself get out of pain. I once again suggested a colon cleanse and explained how her toxic colon might be the cause of her muscles' failure to respond to treatment. She finally took my advice and did the cleanse. I had been treating her for 18 months with poor results, but within three months of doing the colon cleanse, her back was completely healed.

Once her bowels were clear the muscles relaxed and the bones moved easily into alignment and stayed there.

Bones

One might ask why the bones would need to be cleansed. Well, bones are also living tissue. They are not just the bleached white, hardened material we see after they are dried in the sun or cooked. They are actually viable tissue. The wrong type of calcium supplements can create calcium deposits on them. Bones or muscles out of alignment can cause bone spurs or osteoarthritis. A lack of vitamin D, calcium or magnesium can cause bone disease, and toxins can collect in the bones causing tumors or cancer. As discussed in Chapter 10, heavy metals and glyphosate can deposit in the bones, weakening them and acting as a reservoir of toxins. The metal cleansing protocol outlined in that chapter can help clear these things out.

Blood cells are made in the marrow of the bones. The Master Cleanse actually helps to clean out the bones. There are times during a long cleanse (10 days or more) that you will feel your bones ache all over as the cleanse works on them. Soaking in Epsom salts, Cypress and Birch or Wintergreen helps the bones.

I regularly recommend Rehemogen. I feel that it really helps to renew and strengthen bone marrow.

My eldest son had a spiral fracture in his tibia. The orthopedic surgeon told him to elevate his leg and ice it off and on for 10 days, at the end of which period he was going to operate to put screws and a plate in to keep the bone from splintering apart. He did not put a hard cast on it but he did put it in a removable splint, which was fortunate because it allowed us to work on the leg. My husband and I worked on his leg 5 times a day for 5 days. We put Cypress, Wintergreen, Lemongrass, Frankincense, Myrrh, and Idaho Balsam Fir on it each time. We put colloidal silver on it and gave him a teaspoon of colloidal silver to drink every day. We gave him 3000 mg of Calcium, 1500 mg of Magnesium and some vitamin D to take every day. We also gave him 1 teaspoon of Essential Omegas daily. I also used magnets for 5 minutes each session. I rolled the magnets up and down his leg in the direction of the bone after I had applied the silver and oils. Then my husband used a SCENAR device to send electric signals to the brain to boost its involvement in the healing process. My son went back to the doctor on the fifth day of treatment, the 10th day after the accident. We told him to have the doctor X-ray the leg again to see whether it still needed screws and a plate. The doctor was amazed to see that the leg had completely healed! He didn't even put a cast on it. He told my son to use a cane and to begin to put a little bit of weight on it and to do some stretching exercises. After a week, he had complete use of his leg again.

I had another patient who fell 25 feet off the roof of a house and landed on his outstretched arms. He didn't break a bone. As a matter of fact, there were only a few misaligned bones when he came to see me right after it happened. I called his mother and asked her what she fed her son to make his bones so strong. She said that she made sure that he ate well and that he took calcium lactate supplements throughout his growing-up years. He certainly had strong bones!

Teeth

This is a much bigger subject than most people realize, and the teeth can effect many other parts of the body. There a few simple rules I give to my patients about their teeth.

First of all, I recommend that you use a natural toothpaste that is fluoride-free. Despite whatever you may have been taught by the fluoridated-toothpaste industry, fluoride is not necessary for teeth or other bones, and in fact causes a whole host of health problems including mottled teeth, brittle bones, and increased prevalence of hip fractures among the elderly and kidney stones. Toothpaste tubes carry a warning not to swallow toothpaste, and to call the poison control center if you do.

I think most people would be shocked to know that fluoride is the sole ingredient in some rat poisons. So if fluoride is dangerous to swallow, and it kills other mammals that swallow it, why put it in your mouth, where it is absorbed much more quickly than it is in the digestive tract?

Use a toothpaste that isn't contaminated with toxic fluoride. Dentarome, Dentarome Ultra and Dentarome Plus from Young Living Essential Oils are free of fluoride and contain essential oils that will kill microorganisms.

One mother brought in her little girl of about 18 months to me to get her spine adjusted. I noticed that two of the child's lower molars had large cavities in them. I mentioned to her mother that I had heard that Thieves oil could kill the bacteria that cause decay and advised her to use an eyedropper to put one drop of Thieves oil into each cavity three times a day. One week later at her next appointment, the child's teeth looked like new. Amazingly, the dark color of the cavities seemed to have completely disappeared and the teeth looked much improved.

A friend who was having long-term trouble with a tooth rubbed Clove oil on her gums for a few weeks. The next time she saw her dentist her gums were so much improved he asked what she had done to fix it. When she told him about the clove essential oil, he said he had been taught something about clove oil in dental college but had given it no regard—until then.

My own dentist used clove oil on me when I was a child to promote healing, keep down infections and prevent dry socket.

I have heard of others using Clove oil to numb gums for baby teething problems. I have used Lavender for teething with great results, even on older children.

One of my teenage sons whose molars were erupting complained of swollen gums and pain. I had my office in the home at that time and he kept knocking on the door to tell me his teeth and gums hurt. I told him each time to put Lavender on it, but he didn't want to. Finally I got tired of it and excused myself from my patients. I had his older brother tackle him and pry open his mouth as I smeared Lavender oil on his gums. Fifteen minutes later, he came knocking on the door of my office again, but this time he popped his head in and proclaimed, "It worked!"

Cassia essential oil is said to be good for cleaning up the arterial plaque that causes arteriosclerosis. A brave patient discovered that it also cleans plaque off teeth! It is a 'hot' oil—like cinnamon—but within one week it had removed all the plaque from her teeth and her receding gums had returned to normal.

Brain

"Clean the brain? What do you mean clean the brain?" Many people complain about brain fog, inability to think clearly or memory loss. So why not clean the brain? Once again, cleansing the colon and liver, followed by the Master Cleanse and/or a yeast cleanse does wonders for the brain just as it does for the rest of the body. When yeast grows, it emits a gas similar to formaldehyde. Imagine having that on the brain! Try taking Purification oil by mouth and see if that doesn't clear the brain enough to start thinking better. Clarity blend, Brain Power blend and Present Time blend together or separately have proven effective with my patients in clearing the brain.

I once had a group of patients come and discuss their elderly mother with me. They were afraid that she might be getting Alzheimer's and wondered what they could do to help her. We put her on a cleanse, got rid of her yeast infection, gave her Clarity blend and Ningxia Red and all her symptoms disappeared within a few weeks!

I am convinced from my own experience in raising my children, working with patients and involvement with youth groups, that too much sugar has a truly detrimental effect on children. Every mother knows that Easter Sunday, with its traditional baskets of chocolates and other candy, is a day of children bouncing off the walls. I personally feel that if parents would clean up their children's diets and limit sweets, hyperactivity would all but disappear.

After we changed our diets and cut out sugar in my family, my father commented that my children had changed from bouncing off the walls to being able to sit quietly and read books for hours. That change in my children inspired him to change his own diet and start eating healthier foods.

Caffeine too has been shown to decrease blood circulation in the brain. According to a study done by Wake Forest University School of Medicine, the average U.S. daily consumption of caffeine, the equivalent of just over two cups of coffee per day, constricts blood vessels in the brain and causes a reduction in cerebral blood flow. Clearly, maintaining adequate blood flow by avoiding caffeine would be one good way to keep the brain clear.

Essential oils are wonderful for brain function; they are able to go through the blood-brain barrier and carry oxygen to the brain. Another wonderful source of brain food is Essential Omegas. Omega 3-rich fatty acids, such as fish oil and flax seed oil, are indeed essential to nourish the brain, as the brain is made of lipid (fat) material.

Some medical doctors have begun giving flax seed oil to women in their last month of pregnancy because they find that it prevents "post partum blues." The theory is that the baby's brain is rapidly growing during the last month of pregnancy and needs essential fatty acids. If the mother doesn't supply the baby with those needs through her diet, the placenta will take what it needs for the baby from the mother, depleting her of the brain nutrients she needs and leading to depression.

The Limbic System

The limbic system of the brain houses the nerve centers for the emotions and also the organs. When an oil is inhaled, it travels up the 1st cranial nerve to the limbic system of the brain. There are no synapses in that pathway, meaning that inhaled aromas go directly to the brain. The hypothalamus and amygdala are also part of the limbic system. It is through these two small brain organs that all functions of the body are regulated. Essential oils create a chemical effect in that part of the brain that can immediately affect systems throughout the body. An illustration in Appendix F shows this pathway.

A study done by Dr. Terry Freidmann, an MD from Scottsdale, AZ measured the effect of essential oil aromas on brain waves. A young boy, diagnosed with ADHD was wired to an EEG (brain wave monitoring) machine. I saw a video of this experiment, showing the levels of various brain waves on a computer screen.

The amazing thing was that the screen showed mostly Delta and Theta waves, yet the boy was wide awake. Delta and Theta waves are the brain waves that accompany deep sleep! The doctor put a drop of Brain Power on a cotton ball and held it up to the boy's nose for him to breathe. Almost instantly, the brainwaves changed to the more appropriate Beta waves of a person who is awake.

No wonder the boy couldn't focus or do his schoolwork—the thinking part of his brain was asleep. Could this be the answer to the riddle of ADD? Many of my patients now tape a cotton ball with a few drops of Brain Power on it, to their children's chests under their shirts before they go to school. They are seeing remarkable improvements in learning and also a decrease in hyperactivity symptoms.

REFERENCES

Essential Oils Desk Reference 3rd ed., Essential Science Publishing USA 2004

Guyton, Arthur C. Textbook of Medical Physiology. W.B. Saunders Company. Philadelphia PA. 1991

Geofrey Nochimson, MD, Fluoride Toxicity, eMedicine from WebMD, http://www.emedicine.com/emerg/topic181.htm

New England Journal of Medicine, 32, #12, (1990):802-09

Journal of the American Medical Association, 1990-1995 (4 studies on fluoride-related hip fractures)

Rochlitz, Steven, Allergies and Candida, Human Ecology Balancing Sciences, New York NY 1989

Field MD, PhD Aaron S. et al, "Dietary Caffeine Consumption and Withdrawal: Confounding Variables in Quantitative Cerebral Perfusion Studies." Radiology, April 2003

Becker, Robert O., M.D. and Gary Selden. The Body Electric. Morrow. New York. 1985

Morter, Dr. Ted Jr., Dynamic Health. Morter Health Systems. Rogers, Ark 1995

CHAPTER 14

Sick and Tired of Being Sick and Tired

This chapter discusses the various types of chronic fatigue conditions, including Chronic Fatigue Syndrome, Fibromyalgia, Epstein-Barr Syndrome, Anemias, Hypoglycemia and Lupus.

Chronic Fatigue Syndrome

Chronic Fatigue Syndrome (CFS) may arise from any number of underlying disorders, the main symptom being, of course, chronic fatigue. The word 'chronic' here implies a condition that continues over time, i.e. 'continuous fatigue.'

Underlying disorders of, or precursors to CFS may include adrenal insufficiency, thyroid disorders, (both discussed in Chapter 15), yeast infections (Chapter 7), lupus, various anemias and others. Usually if a person has one of these disorders he/she has many if not all of the other precursors for CFS, so when treating CFS we really need to treat for all of the related diseases. CFS's symptoms may include indigestion, upper and lower gas, poor assimilation, poor electrolyte balance, allergic reaction to food and other substances, mood swings, fatigue, irritability, and a lack of motivation, discipline and creativity. This is by no means an exhaustive list.

It is very important to have a complete physical exam if you think you have CFS to help rule out any of the above as underlying causes. It is extremely important to have a complete history taken because some diseases such as lupus have symptoms that come and go through the years and may not always be present at the same time. Good lab work is also important. (However, sometimes organ malfunction isn't severe enough to show up on blood lab tests. In these cases, although the condition may be real, it is sub-clinical, and conventional medicine does not treat sub-clinical problems.)

The examining doctor should look at various types of anemia, including B vitamin deficiency, iron deficiency, hemolytic anemia etc. Parasitic infestations should be considered. The possibility of *candida albicans* overgrowth should be checked by means of stool samples and also dark-field microscopy to see whether it has infiltrated the blood. A comprehensive review of symptoms can uncover nutritional or hormonal deficiencies.

In our clinic, the usual starting point for treating all the diseases that underlie CFS is the same, since they are all interrelated. You guessed it...we start with a colon cleanse and a liver cleanse.

We might do a yeast cleanse if needed, or the Master Cleanse (See Chapter 2 for an understanding of the best order in which to cleanse.) We add nutritional support to the adrenals, thyroid, pancreas and hormonal systems. We treat any underlying viral or bacterial infections. In my office we determine on an individual basis which systems to treat and in what order.

Yeast or candida albicans is a major cause of chronic fatigue and fibromyalgia. To learn more about this problem, see Chapter 7, which is dedicated entirely to yeast cleansing.

The following are some of the more common and serious symptoms related to chronic fatigue, along with treatment recommendations: (Treatment of the thyroid and adrenal glands, which are also major players in CFS, are discussed in Chapter 15.)

Fibromyalgia

Fibromyalgia is a type of CFS characterized by severe muscle pain in the neck and shoulders. Fibromyalgia literally means muscle pain of unknown origin, and sometimes it is truly a mystery where it comes from.

Many who suffer from fibromyalgia have a thyroid component to their illness. Sometimes just treating them for hypothyroidism takes care of the fibromyalgia. I have also had patients with a medical diagnosis of fibromyalgia who had herniated discs in their necks and once that was corrected the pain disappeared. Some people are just plain toxic or have candida overgrowth. Many times simply doing a colon cleanse followed by the Master Cleanse takes care of the toxicity in the joints and the pain decreases.

One of my patients whose medical doctor gave her a diagnosis of fibromyalgia finally figured out that the pain in her shoulders started about the same time she started having her nails sculptured at a nail shop. The fumes from the chemicals used there and the products that remained on her fingernails for weeks afterward were causing a toxic liver reaction, sending pain (and possibly the toxins themselves) to her shoulders. She quit going to the nail studio, I put her on a liver cleanse and that was the end of her fibromyalgia.

Different anti-inflammatory oils may alleviate the symptoms of fibromyalgia while treating the cause. Clove and Nutmeg essential oils and Regenolone Cream have corticosteroid activity. They often do a great job of reducing inflammation in joints caused by arthritic conditions such as rheumatoid or lupus arthritis. Aroma Seiz blend, Marjoram, Relieve It, Raindrop Technique, Release, Idaho Balsam Fir and Lavender all help with muscle pain or spasm. You will probably have to experiment with the different oils to discover which one your body responds to best.

Epstein-Barr

Epstein-Barr is a virus that can cause chronic fatigue. It is believed to be similar to the virus responsible for mononucleosis. Signs of a "mono" infection include fever, sore throat, headaches, white patches on the back of the throat, swollen glands in the neck, tiredness and lack of appetite.

The virus is supposed to go away on its own within about 4 weeks, and in most cases that is what happens. However, some feel that this same virus is also responsible for long-term fatigue that could last years. Others think that the virus harbors in the spine and can cause scoliosis.

The virus is often easy to treat by doing Raindrop technique on the spine a couple of times a week and taking one 00 capsule a day of diluted Thieves blend, Oregano, Thyme or Mountain Savory essential oils, until the symptoms have disappeared.

Anemias

There are many types of anemia that cause fatigue. Low iron is probably the most common. Iron is the component of red blood cells that carries oxygen to the cells. If the level of iron in the blood is low the cells cannot get the oxygen they need to carry on their metabolism and catabolism functions.

In women the most common cause of iron-poor blood is heavy bleeding during childbirth, miscarriage or menstrual periods. The solution, obviously, is to rebuild the stores of iron in the body. Blackstrap molasses is an easily digested source of iron. Yellow dock and dandelion root are also good sources of iron, but it takes several months to build up iron levels using these herbal teas. Some people take chlorophyll drinks regularly to build the blood.

A quick source of iron is to eat liver 3 times a day for 3 straight days—if you can stand to do that.

Here is a better solution: Rehemogen from Young Living Essential Oils. It's a great blood builder. 'Re' means again, 'heme' means blood and 'gen' means genesis, so the name well describes this product, which rebuilds blood. I have seen it quickly rebuild the blood of a female patient who had anemeia due to a serious hemorrhage.

Of course this advice is directed primarily to women. Men may want to build their blood too if not getting enough iron in the diet, but a man who has unusually low iron and cannot attribute it to serious blood loss from an injury of some kind, may well be be suffering from some kind of internal bleeding, as in the case of colon cancer. A man who is severely anemic should immediately see a medical doctor.

A lack of B vitamins (specifically B-12 and folic acid) can cause pernicious anemia. The word 'pernicious' in this case implies life threatening. Not only is the person tired but he or she will have difficulty with digestion. Once again, this is easy to remedy through diet modification. In this case eating a lot of dark leafy green foods. Vitagreen helps build the B-vitamins. Super-B from Young Living is one of the best B vitamin supplements that I have seen. Blackstrap molasses is a good source of B vitamins, as is liver. Any of the nervine class of herbs is also a good source of B vitamins.

Hemolytic anemia is a serious condition in which the red blood cells break up and spill their iron. Those with this condition can suddenly become extremely tired and their limbs will hurt, then start to ache. Sometimes they become feverish. The fever is a result of the bone marrow heating up to make new red blood cells. This occurs frequently in lupus patients. Again, Rehemogen is excellent for rebuilding the blood and helping the bone marrow produce new red blood cells.

I recommend Rehemogen in any flu or feverish condition as it will support the bone marrow while it is making white or red blood cells.

Hypoglycemia

Hypoglycemia is a condition in which the blood glucose (sugar) level drops below the correct range. It might spike or rise very rapidly followed by a sharp drop or it may drop off slowly but continue to decline below normal levels. When blood glucose drops this low, a person may experience severe headache, stomach pain or nausea, or may suddenly become tired and need to take a nap. Often people with hypoglycemia experience anger and sudden temper outbursts. They may have an intense appetite that makes them feel like they are starving.

These incidents are often provoked by their consumption of simple sugars found in candy and high starch, sugary foods without some protein to balance them.

A person with hypoglycemia should avoid any food that converts quickly into sugar, including processed foods and starches. Complex carbohydrates take longer to digest and are easier on the body, but even these can create a problem if they are not balanced with protein. Hypoglycemia generally stems from a liver that is not digesting sugars properly, but it can also arise from pancreatic imbalances. Viruses, parasites, yeast or other microorganisms may be contributing factors.

Doctors generally treat the symptoms of hypoglycemia by telling the patient to eat several small meals a day and not to let the stomach go empty. The hypoglycemic is told to watch what he or she eats and to limit intake of simple sugars.

Some people will try to balance a sweet juice or a candy bar with some kind of protein hoping to prevent low blood sugar, but that generally starts the body into a vicious cycle of spiked blood sugar followed by low blood sugar.

Here is what I recommend:

For symptomatic relief, ¼ cup of NingXia Red juice blend will usually raise the blood sugar in about 15-20 minutes, and will relieve the headache, nausea, shakiness and fatigue caused by a low glucose level.

If the problem originates in the pancreas, Sulferzyme taken according to directions and 3 drops of stevia extract every day generally corrects the pancreatic imbalance in a couple of weeks.

If the problem is in the liver, Essentialzymes-4 capsules and a liver cleanse (See Chapter 9) will correct the problem.

Of course if the problem is caused by a microorganism, the specific type of infection must be addressed. See specific recommendations related to yeast, parasites, viruses and bacteria discussed elsewhere in this book.

Diet has a lot to do with hypoglycemia. Nutritionist Barry Sears, PhD, has authored an excellent book called <u>The Omega Zone</u> that discusses the relationship between food and the sugar hormones of the body and how to keep things in balance through diet modification. I highly recommend his book to anyone who wants to learn how to eat in a healthy, balanced way.

Lupus

Lupus is an exasperating (and sometimes terrifying) condition as it can mimic every disease in the book, yet no treatment seems to work. I have personally suffered with lupus for several years, so I know how challenging this condition can be.

People who have chronic fatigue that is not responding to any of the above treatment plans may actually have lupus. In that case, all of the problems discussed above turn out not to be causes of chronic fatigue but symptoms of lupus. It is still necessary to treat all these problems to help control the pain and fatigue of lupus, but it is also necessary to treat the cause of the lupus itself, which can be a very difficult thing to do as it is an autoimmune disease.

That means that the immune system itself is incorrectly identifying healthy tissue as a foreign invader in the body. This causes normally protective forces within the body to attack itself.

It is generally thought that overproduction of histamines by the mast cells is the cause of the inflammation characteristic of lupus. The thymus gland is responsible for controlling this inflammatory process of the body. It is a delicate thing to treat inflammation in a lupus patient because if treatment is too vigorous the immune system becomes over-stimulated and provokes a flare-up of lupus symptoms, which is what you were trying to decrease in the first place.

It is very important for lupus patients to keep their bodies in balance and to maintain good colon and liver health. They need to keep the pH of the body in balance and support their body systems with good nutrition and extra supplementation.

A study in Japan followed over 600 lupus patients to observe the long term prognosis of the disease and to check the possibility of achieving long term remission. Most of the patients were treated with steroids and chemotherapy to decrease the immune response. Because only 17 of the patients achieved long term remission, the researchers concluded that it was almost impossible to achieve long term remission from lupus.

But on closer examination it was discovered that out of the 17 patients that had gone into remission, 13 had refused all medical treatment! That was an amazing finding. It told me if a lupus patient wants to have any chance of remission from lupus symptoms, the best hope is to <u>forego the medical route!</u>

We have had several patients achieve relief from their symptoms enough to function in a fairly normal lifestyle. We are still working on a natural remedy for lupus using Frankincense and Sandalwood essential oils along with energy and emotional release techniques, to gain long term relief of symptoms.

In my own case, I have had much better results using essential oils than I ever got using herbs and glandular extracts.

Lupus is diagnosed primarily by a history of symptoms, since only 50 percent of the people who have lupus have lupus markers in their blood.

Making positive diagnosis even more difficult, There is such a thing as 'pseudo-lupus,' in which a person has lupus symptoms arising simply from excess toxicity in the body. These individuals sometimes experience seemingly miraculous "lupus cures" when they do a cleanse or take nutritional supplements that supply what they had been missing.

Lupus symptoms can include:

- Extreme fatigue
- Painful or swollen joints (arthritis)
- Muscle pain and stiffness
- Unexplained fever
- Skin rashes
- Kidney problems
- Hair loss
- Nausea, vomiting, abdominal pain
- Headaches, migraines,
- Seizures
- Strokes and transient ischemic attacks (TIA)

- Depression, anxiety, confusion
- Photosensitivity (sensitivity to sunlight)
- Skin thickening (scleroderma), ligament breakage
- Vasculitis (swelling of veins and arteries)
- Nephritis (Kidney swelling)
- Hemolytic Anemia (breakage of red blood cells with resultant loss of iron)
- Pleurisy

Tests which help to confirm a lupus diagnosis:
- Complete blood count
- Erythrocyte sedimentation rate (ESR)—an elevated ESR indicates inflammation in the body
- Urinalysis
- Blood chemistries
- Complement test (a blood test that measures severity of infection)
- Antinuclear antibody test (ANA)—positive in most lupus patients; other antibody tests
- Syphilis test (may be falsely positive in people with lupus)
- Skin or kidney biopsy

Nutritional tips for patients with lupus include the following:
- Eliminate all suspected allergens, including dairy, wheat (gluten), soy, chocolate, eggs, corn, and preservatives; avoid alfalfa sprouts. Your healthcare provider may want to test for food sensitivities.
- A modified fast of five to seven days at two-week intervals may be helpful, especially during flare-ups. A modified fast can consist of eating fruits, vegetables, and limiting protein to fish or vegetable protein.
- Avoid coffee, alcohol, and smoking.
- Minimize red meat and saturated fats to decrease inflammation. Avoid pork products entirely.

Potentially beneficial nutrient supplements for those with lupus include the following:
- Omega-3 fatty acids such as flaxseed and fish oils to decrease inflammation.
- Beta-carotene (50 mg three times a day), although some controversy exists about the use of vitamin A. Check with your health care provider before using.
- Vitamin B12 (1,000 mcg via injection once or twice a week) to heal lesions.
- Vitamin E (800 IU per day)
- Hydrochloric acid (Betaine HCl) to decrease symptoms.
- DHEA (start at 5 mg three times a day and work up to 100 mg per day) to reduce symptoms in mild to moderate lupus.

- Note: Tryptophan should be avoided in patients with SLE-type lupus.
- Melatonin (2-3 mg before bed) has been shown to be helpful in many autoimmune diseases. Take a lower dose if drowsiness occurs.
- Methylsulfonylmethane (MSM) (up to 3,000 mg twice a day) helps prevent joint and connective tissue breakdown.
- Iron can increase inflammation. Avoid artificial iron supplements.

The following is a list of various lupus symptoms and what we have used to treat them naturally:

- Seizures: Sandalwood, Frankincense, Valerian essential oils and Peace and Calming blend via foot reflexology or a drop in the cheek.
- Hives: Australian Blue, Lavender and Ningxia Red juice blend; also increase zinc
- Vasculitis (swollen veins): Australian Blue and Idaho Balsam Fir mixed together and applied topically on the back of the hand. A drop may also be taken in the cheek. This usually brings the swelling down quickly.
- Joint Swelling: Nutmeg and Clove essential oils and Regenolone cream, applied topically
- Photosensitivity (eyes and skin): zinc
- Trigeminal neuralgia (pain in face and behind and on top of ears): Frankincense and Lemongrass essential oils, applied topically
- Migraines: foot reflexology with any essential oil, (I start with Valor) or the oils for seizures above; some people get results by putting 3-4 drops of Peppermint, PanAway, or M-grain in their hands, rubbing them together, then cupping them over mouth and nose and breathing it until the headache subsides.
- Nephritis (swelling of kidney): K&B extract, Sage, Rosemary, Ledum, Idaho Balsam Fir in compresses; Juniper orally; acupuncture; 1-3 drops of Geranium in water a few times a day.
- Hypothyroidism: Endoflex blend, Sclaressence
- Hypoadrenia: nutmeg essential oil, Super B, Mineral Essence, Sclaressence, DHEA
- Pleurisy (swelling of lung lining): breathe in steam, Thyme, Peppermint, RC blend, Australian Blue blend, and Lavender. Marshmallow root also helps pleurisy
- Yeast: Melrose blend, Stevia extract, Australian Blue blend, Probiotics

(see Chapter 7 for more on yeast)

- Nutrient assimilation: Polyzyme or other enzymes as needed
- Skin outbreaks: Lavender, soaking in Epsom Salts and Clove (See the section on skin cleansing in Chapter 10)
- Hormonal Imbalances: Progesterone cream, Sclaressence (see Chapter on Hormones)
- Parasites: Parafree
- Viruses: Raindrop technique, a 00 capsule of of Oregano diluted 50-50 in olive oil, nightly
- pH imbalance: Vitagreen, Master Cleanse periodically,
- keep colon and digestion functioning with frequent cleanses.
- Emotions to work on: Intolerance of self, forgiveness of self, acceptance of self. It is important to keep stress to a minimum as it can cause a flare-up. Use Peace and Calming, Valor and Forgiveness blends, meditation and relaxation techniques.
- To work on a genetic cause, use Frankincense, Sandalwood and Three Wise Men. Have a trusted partner or professional do energy work or work with the scripts from Carol Truman's book, *Feelings Buried Alive Never Die.*

The critical issue in treating lupus is that you must keep the body in balance. It requires the patient's constant attention. Stress, parasites, hormonal imbalances, pregnancy and viruses all cause flares. Stress is especially likely to cause flares. Keep sugar to a minimum, eat naturally and balance carbs and proteins, keep the liver and colon clean especially during allergy seasons, get plenty of rest and support your organs nutritionally. Acid buildup is said to increase the likelihood of autoimmune conditions, causing antibodies to attack the body instead of bacteria and other foreign invaders, so keep the body alkalized. Forgiveness oil, Frankincense, Cedarwood, Sandalwood, Myrrh, Onchya, and Idaho Balsam Fir help to protect DNA. Lupus symptoms may stem from the genetic defect MTHFR (see Chapter 18).

It is very important to find and consult with a doctor who understands how to treat for chronic fatigue syndrome and its relatives, because in many cases—with proper treatment—a patient may become sicker before they get better. The doctor can give advice on how to pull through the rough times. Also, individual treatment plans can be formulated around how much of each product to use and when to start with each product.

There are additional techniques that can be taught to the patient to help alleviate the pain and discomfort that sometimes occurs while cleansing. It is important to find a doctor who can do organ manipulation and can take energy blocks off the body's nervous system. In addition to essential oils, consider chiropractic, acupuncture, energy balancing and emotional release techniques.

Some of the emotions connected with specific lupus symptoms are:
- Yeast --- frustration or feeling overwhelmed
- Hypoglycemia --- missing the sweetness in life, or the sweetness has disappeared in your life
- Hypoadrenia --- sick and tired of being sick and tired
- Lupus --- inability to forgive or accept one's self

Louise Hay's book <u>Heal Your Body</u> has a complete list of different disease states and the emotions that go with them. If you have lupus, I recommend you consult her book in addition to following the steps outlined above.

Case History #1

One day when my daughter, Heather was about 15 years old, I found her in her room standing frozen, staring into space, completely unable to function. She stayed in bed for several weeks missing school, crying and sleeping intermittently. I took her to my medical doctor, but he couldn't tell us what was wrong. He suggested counseling for emotional problems. For the next several years she struggled, but beginning when she was 21 her condition degenerated to the point that she became virtually incapacitated and had to quit a job she loved working as a counselor for a wilderness survival program.

I decided to try an MD-turned-naturopathic doctor. He diagnosed Chronic Fatigue Syndrome and Fibromyalgia, but the medicine he prescribed could only be used for 6 months. During those 6 months she improved about 20 percent, but immediately after her prescription ran out she was worse than ever. By that time her condition was so bad she was sleeping 12-14 hours a day, was suffering from chronic gastric distress, constant body aches and pains, upper respiratory infections and severe cognitive dysfunction. Unable to go to school, work, or pursue her exceptional singing talent, she spent the bulk of her time, when she wasn't in bed, lying on the sofa watching movies.

I began applying essential oils on Heather twice daily when she was 23 years old. One month later, on December 15th, the family made a two-day trip to St. Louis. Usually Heather was a bear to travel with, sleeping every minute in the car except for an occasional grouchy potty stop. Much to our amazement, however, on this trip, we were delighted to note that Heather actually stayed awake much of the time and participated in conversation. That was the beginning of a miraculous change.

In another month Heather was staying awake more and more. By February of 2001, I almost cried when I saw her doing her own laundry. Soon she found a job that required only 10 hours a week, which allowed her to transition into "normal life." In a couple of months the job turned into a full time job. A few months after that she found out that there was a new wilderness survival program in Utah. Anxiously wondering whether she could handle the rigors of the wilderness again, she applied. She got the job immediately and worked there for a about two years as a counselor for troubled youth. She hiked 4-6 miles a day, carried a 30-40 lb pack on her back, and was responsible for 6-10 troubled youth day and night for 8 days in a row with a week off before the next stint. In the meantime she would apply the oils intermittently. Eventually she completed a "triple," which is three 8-day shifts in a row, meaning that for 24 straight days she worked in the wilderness, and much to everyone's joy, she did fine.

Still using the essential oils intermittently, Heather has served as an LDS missionary, has married, and given birth to a beautiful baby girl. She is remodelling a home and is healthy and happy. But that isn't the only essential oil miracle I have witnessed. Through applying the oils to Heather, the oils absorbed into my skin as well. Over a period of 3 months I realized my chronic leg, hip, and ankle pain that I had suffered from for more than a decade had disappeared. I could walk, sit, and sleep without pain. I also realized that my memory, and especially my college vocabulary, had all returned. My mind was sharp and clear like it had not been since I was in my twenties. I felt like a new woman.

I have been blessed twice, first with a healthy, productive daughter, and second, with a pain-free life full of hope for the future.

Coleen Gleason
Orem Utah

Case History #2

Beth came to see me after her fourth miscarriage. The first thing I noticed was the lupus butterfly mask on her face. She showed me her blood work that she had recently had done with a medical doctor. She had the typical systemic lupus erythematosis (SLE) markers in her blood and was diagnosed with SLE. Her medical doctor told her that the reason she had miscarriages was that the body was attacking and killing the fetuses. She asked me if she could ever get pregnant and keep the baby. I told her that it was certainly worth a try. I put her on the regime outlined in this book. I also asked her if she experienced the emotions that go with lupus. Those emotions are hatred of self, unforgiveness of self, beating one's self up and wishing she were dead. She said that she did have those emotions. I asked her whether she laid awake at night beating herself up for things she had done or said during the day. She said that she did. I put her on Valor, Joy, Peace and Calming and Forgiveness essential oil blends. I told her to use those oil blends several times a day. I told her that whenever she started to mentally "beat herself up" she was to smell the Forgiveness oil and to repeat 10 times, "I love and forgive myself. I choose forgiveness of myself and others, I am a wonderful, worthwhile person. Life is precious to me."

After two months, her husband came to visit me and wanted to know if it was worth the expense of the supplements. I told him to stay with it for 6 months and if she wasn't better or pregnant in that time they could quit. I asked him if it would be worth it if she had a baby. He said that it most definitely would be worth all that he had. Two months later she came to me with a new blood report. All the lupus markers were gone from her blood. Her doctor was amazed since he had never seen that happen in all his years of medical practice. Her butterfly mask was gone from her face. She had strength and energy. She loved herself and all around her. More importantly she was expecting again and was 2 months pregnant. The last time I talked to Beth she had had three beautiful girls in a 4 year time span. She was well, loving life and a lifelong fan of Young Living Essential Oils.

REFERENCES

Guyton, Arthur C. Textbook of Medical Physiology. W.B. Saunders Company. Philadelphia PA. 1991 Bested, Alison, M.D. and Alan C. Logan. Hope and Help for Chronic Fatigue Syndrome and Fibromyalgia. Cumberland House Publishing.2006

St. Amand, R.Paul. M.D., and Claudia Craig Marek and Mair Florence. What your Doctor May not Tell you About Fibromyalgia. Warner Books. New York. NY. 1999

Crook, William G., The Yeast Connection: A Medical Breakthrough. Random House. New York, NY. 1986

Trowbridge, John P., MD., and Dr. Morton Walker. The Yeast Syndrome. Bantam Books. New York, NY. 1986

Randolph, Theron G., MD. and Ralph W. Moss Ph.D., An Alternative Approach to Allergies. Harper &Row. New York, NY.1989

Martin, Jeanne Marie. Complete Candida Yeast Guidebook. Prima Publishing. CA. 2000

Beers, Mark H., M.D., and Robert Berkow, M.D., The Merck Manual, Merck and Co., Inc. 2005

Walther, David S. Applied Kinesiology Synopsis. Systems DC. Pueblo, CO 1988

Lupus Foundation of America, www.lupus.org

Hay, Louise. Heal Your body. Hay House, Inc. Carlsbad, CA. 1984

CHAPTER 15

Pituitary, Thyroid, Adrenals: Glands That Make You Go

The endocrine system of the body includes many glands. These include the pituitary, thyroid and adrenal glands, the reproductive glands—the ovaries, uterus, and testes—and the pineal, parathyroid and thymus. What the endocrine glands all have in common is the production of hormones to direct the metabolic functions of the body. The placenta also produces certain hormones

Although each gland produces its own particular hormone(s), they all affect each other either directly or through feedback mechanisms. Additionally, as has been discussed in previous chapters, the adrenals produce some sex hormones, and the liver constantly removes excess hormones of all types. This complex interrelationship of the endocrine glands and indeed all the systems of the body is what often makes diagnoses difficult. A hormone imbalance can sometimes mimic a nervous breakdown. It can also contribute to chronic fatigue. In this chapter we will discuss the three glands that direct energy usage in the body: the pituitary, the thyroid and the adrenals.

The pituitary gland is the often called the master gland of the body. Its purpose is to send hormonal signals to the other glands to direct them to produce their respective hormones. It also produces important direct-acting hormones. The thyroid regulates metabolism, while the adrenal glands produce hormones to assist the body with energy production as well as other functions. These three glands are the energy trio, and other than the sex glands (discussed in Chapter 16), are the ones that most often need support.

Remember as you do the cleanses or use the procedures that are mentioned in this chapter that it generally takes 3-4 months before you notice a big change in hormone production. Keep using the products for at least that long. Some people notice a change immediately but others notice more gradual improvement. Most people, however, find that their hormonal difficulties are cleared up within 4 months.

Let us start with the master gland of the body and find out what its functions are and how to assist it in functioning properly. Be aware, though, that all these glands are adversely affected by chemicals in our food and environment (such as glyphosate, found in genetically modified plants), so we must first take care to avoid them.

The pituitary gland

The pituitary gland gets its orders from the hypothalamus, which acts as a sort of interface between the nervous system and the endocrine system. The pituitary then sends hormonal signals to the other endocrine glands directing them to produce their respective hormones or to send out signals to other glands, and it produces several hormones that have a direct effect as well. One of these is human growth hormone (HGH). The pituitary also sends signals to the ovaries or testes, to the kidneys to control water retention, to the uterus to promote contraction at the time of childbirth, and to the mammary glands to produce milk after childbirth.

If the pituitary as the master gland of the body is not functioning correctly, the other glands and organs will not function correctly. When dealing with difficult cases of infertility or hormonal imbalances or chronic fatigue it is important to check the function of the pituitary gland. It can become inflamed during a hemorrhage or a miscarriage, or the bones in the head (particularly the sphenoid bone) may for some reason create pressure on the turça sellica, which houses the pituitary gland. If this is the case, first see a craniopath, generally a chiropractor who has specialized in moving cranial bones, to relieve the pressure on the gland.

Sometimes instead of functioning normally the pituitary will produce adenomas, which are hormone-filled sacs, leading to symptoms that mimic hypothyroidism. The symptoms of an adenoma can creep up on a person slowly. It might start with slight hormone imbalances or slight fatigue, and as the sac or adenoma grows the symptoms worsen. It can lead to severe frontal or migraine headaches and worsening fatigue to the point of exhaustion and the need to sleep 12-15 hours a day. If a person is having severe headaches daily, especially frontal and between the eyes, or semihemipelegic migraines (pain, numbness, a burning sensation or paralysis on one side of the body), he or she should go to a doctor to be checked for an adenoma of the pituitary gland.

If a pituitary adenoma is found it can easily be dissolved using Ultra Young + spray. Usually I tell people to spray the spray twice into each cheek 4 times a day. Use the spray for 4 months to make sure that the pituitary gland is balanced and functioning correctly again. It also helps to put a drop of Frankincense and a drop of Lavender oil on the roof of the mouth 4-5 times a day. Even if you don't have an adenoma, but you do have a hypopituitary condition, use the Ultra Young + spray. In both cases use the spray for a minimum of 4 months to make sure that you have changed the tissue.

Gigantism and dwarfism stem from abnormalities in the pituitary production of HGH. I have used Ultra Young + spray for both conditions and have seen wonderful results.

Thyroid

Under the direction of the pituitary, the thyroid sends hormones, primarily thyroxin, that boost the metabolism of practically every cell in the body, approximately doubling the body's rate of activity. This includes the other endocrine glands; thus if the thyroid doesn't send out the correct amount of thyroxin to the other endocrine glands they won't produce their hormones properly. The thyroid may malfunction in being either under- or over-active. The more common condition is an under-active thyroid, called hypothyroidism. Hypothyroidism is one cause of chronic fatigue syndrome, which was discussed in Chapter 14. When the thyroid is underactive it can cause profound fatigue. The sufferer simply does not want to get up and do anything. It is possible to have mild fatigue in the beginning stages of hypothyroidism but as it worsens the person gets more and more tired each day. Many people complain of major depression or mental issues, not realizing that they have hypothyroidism, and after a visit to a medical doctor end up spending the rest of their lives on anti-depressant medications. Several patients have said that they feel like they are living in a box in their head, screaming to get out of it. They feel like banging their head on a wall to relieve the pressure in the head. This is a sign that they may have not only hypothyroidism but a problem with the pituitary gland as well.

Symptoms of hypothyroidism include:

- Fatigue
- Weakness
- Weight gain or increased difficulty losing weight
- Coarse, dry hair
- Dry, rough pale skin
- Hair loss
- Cold intolerance (can't tolerate the cold like most people in the same environment)
- Muscle cramps and frequent muscle aches
- Constipation
- Depression
- Irritability
- Memory loss
- Abnormal menstrual cycles
- Decreased libido
- Hormonal imbalances

These symptoms may or may not all be present. Some may be milder than others. Sometimes a blood test will point to hypothyroidism, while other times if the problem is still sub-clinical, the blood test will come back normal. But the problem is still real! Unfortunately, conventional medicine does not recognize sub-clinical diseases. This is where alternative medicine comes to the rescue.

There are many different causes of hypothyroidism, including inflammation, nodules, and hypo-pituitarism, but hypothyroidism is fairly easy to treat. We begin by jumpstarting Endoflex oil. (See Chapter 3 on how to use essential oils). The thyroid also loves Myrtle oil. Myrtle oil is found in Endoflex but sometimes I also have a patient use more Myrtle in addition to the Endoflex. It's also helpful to rub Endoflex, Lemongrass and Myrtle on the throat. Sometimes people react to Lemongrass and break out in a rash on the throat where it was applied. You could try diluting it to see if you are sensitive that way. Do not put Lemongrass oil directly in the mouth undiluted. It is very hot and will burn and blister the mucous lining of the mouth.

Thyromin is an excellent supplement to feed the Thyroid gland whether it is under- or over-active. Take two Thyromin capsules at night. Some people have found that taking Thyromin at night causes them to have insomnia for a few days. This passes in about 5 days. You can try taking one capsule for a few days and then move up to two or taking it in the morning for a week or two then switching back to night. It is important to take the Thyromin at night because the thyroid receives its major energy from the meridian system between 9 and 11 pm, so taking it then allows the body to use it at the proper time. Remember that it takes about 4 months to change a tissue in the body so do not stop doing your program before that time. You may or may not see instant results. If you do begin to feel better, you must still continue the program for the full 4 months to make sure that you do not backslide and that the tissues have truly healed. If you do not see an immediate improvement, don't be discouraged since it may take the entire 4 months before you see any results.

Sometimes a person also has adrenal insufficiency (see below) in addition to hypothyroidism. In this case, take two Thyromin at night and one in the morning. If you are extremely exhausted, keep adding one Thyromin at night, then one in the morning until you reach a level where your energy rises.

Besides hypothyroidism, a goiter can sometimes cause hyperthyroidism, which is an increase in the body metabolism. A goiter shows up as a swelling around the thyroid. Other things can also cause swelling of the thyroid so it is best to have it checked out by a doctor. A goiter is caused by not getting or absorbing enough iodine, the thyroid swelling in response as it tries to carry out its duties. If you have been diagnosed with goiter, a simple test to see whether you need more iodine is to get some liquid iodine and paint a 2" square patch of your abdomen with it. Check it in 20 minutes. If it has absorbed into the skin and not left a stain, it's an indication that you need more iodine in your system. Repaint an area with iodine. Then check every day to see if there is a stain. If not, repaint with iodine. When your body has all the iodine it needs, the painted iodine will not be absorbed but will instead stain the skin yellow or orange. Generally by then the goiter has disappeared. Most people generally begin staining in a few days, though I have known some people who took several weeks get enough iodine. (Iodine deficiency has been implicated in fibrocystic breast disease, uterine fibroids and other disorders.)

In addition to simply not getting enough iodine in the diet, an iodine insufficiency can result from environmental factors, the most common being chemical pollutants added intentionally to our lives. Fluoride and chlorine from public water supplies and fluoride in toothpaste compete with iodine for the reception sites of the thyroid gland. So does bromine, an ingredient in commercial breads, sports drinks and citrus-flavored soft drinks (and it's especially strong in Mountain Dew). This is because they are all halogen gases, members of group 17 on the periodic table of elements—but iodine is much less reactive than the other halogens. (Fluorine, in fact, is the most reactive of all elements.)

That means that fluorine, chlorine and bromine bind more powerfully than iodine with the same elements or compounds. In the thyroid gland they grab onto the iodine receptor sites, but although these halogens are chemically related to iodine, they do not perform the same functions in the thyroid gland. All they do is make it impossible for the thyroid to get the iodine it requires. I highly recommend that you pay attention to the ingredient list on bread products, and that you get a good filter for your household water supply that will remove the fluorine and the chlorine. It isn't just a problem with drinking water; these gases can also absorb through the skin in bathwater. As a side note, although there are other problems associated with Prozac use, it also contains 30 percent fluorine by weight – not good.

I also recommend that you use a natural toothpaste that is fluoride-free. Despite whatever you may have been taught by the fluoridated-toothpaste industry, fluoride is not necessary for teeth or other bones, and in fact causes a whole host of health problems including mottled teeth, brittle bones, increased prevalence of hip fractures among the elderly, calcification of the pineal gland and kidney stones. The nations of Europe and indeed most of the world refuse to fluoridate their water, for good reason. In fact, fluoride was formerly used to depress thyroid function in hyperthyroidism, and the dose required to achieve this is no more than what we receive in fluoridated water. Permissible levels of fluoride intake were shown to cause brain damage, including a drop in IQ, in a study published in 2014 in the journal Lancet Neurology.

Fluoride is actually a waste product of the aluminum and fertilizer industries and would be an expensive toxic waste problem for these industries if they weren't able to dump it on the public for its phony health benefits. Toothpaste tubes even carry a warning not to swallow toothpaste, and to call the poison control center if you do. By the way, fluoride is the main ingredient in rat poison, or was, until warfarin came along. Professional scoffers say this isn't true, but I have personally seen an old box of rat poison labeled sodium fluoride. Dr. Dean Burk, former head chemist at the National Cancer Institute, said "Fluoridated water is public murder on a grand scale." (Of course this did not refer entirely to thyroid conditions.)

So if it's dangerous to swallow it, why put it in your mouth, where it is absorbed much more quickly than it is in the digestive tract? Use a toothpaste that isn't contaminated with toxic fluoride. Dentrome, Dentrome Ultra and Dentrome Plus from Young Living Essential Oils are free of fluoride and contain essential oils that will kill microorganisms. And, as I said, I also recommend you get a water filter that will remove dangerous chemicals from your drinking and cooking water, and even from bathing water if possible.

Adrenal Glands

The adrenals are very busy glands, producing a whole host of hormones that play a large role in the regulation of body systems. Probably the most well-known is "adrenalin," the real name of which is epinephrine. Adrenalin is what gives the body the energy to "get up and go." It is called the "fight or flight" hormone because the adrenals pump out a lot of it in emergency situations to increase the heart rate, inhibit the activity of the gastro-intestinal tract and otherwise prime the body for action. Adrenalin also helps to control blood pressure, heart rate, sweating, and other activities that are also regulated by the sympathetic nervous system. This hormone is produced in the adrenal medulla along with norepinephrine, which works with epinephrine, and dopamine.

The cortex of the adrenal gland produces hormone building blocks for the reproductive system to create the male and female reproductive hormones. The adrenals also make some reproductive hormones themselves. When a person is having hormonal difficulties it is important to ensure that the adrenal glands are functioning properly, particularly in the case of a male.

Adrenocorticoid hormones are also produced in the adrenal cortex. These include various mineralocorticoids, mostly aldosterone, and glucocorticoids, the most well-known of which is cortisol. Aldosterone's primary role is to promote retention of sodium in the body, which causes retention of water. Without aldosterone we would quickly die of dehydration.

Cortisol is the "stress hormone." It is released under any type of stress. Its main purpose is to break down protein stores to allow the liver to turn protein into glucose rapidly so the brain can have more energy to deal with the stressful situation. The flight or flight mechanism in the body is working on high during times of stress and more energy and blood sugar is consumed. Elevated cortisol can also begin to tear up ligaments between bones causing the spine and joints to go out of alignment easily and frequently, and it can draw protein from bones, leading to osteoporosis. Essentially, cortisol causes the body to scavenge protein from everywhere except the liver, breaking down everything for the sake of glucose for brainpower to deal with the perceived stress. It is also noteworthy that cortisol severely depresses the immune system.

Here are a few examples of stressors that could cause elevated levels of cortisol:

- Excess heat or cold
- Alcohol abuse
- Coffee drinking
- Depression
- Anxiety
- Malnutrition
- Personal relationships
- Physical or emotional trauma
- Surgery
- Job-related problems
- Diseases

The adrenal glands of a person who lives a stress-filled life are constantly creating cortisol in an effort to deal with it and thereby tearing down muscles and bones and depressing the immune system. This person is probably also living in a constant state of fear (perhaps unrecognized), activating the over-production of adrenalin, which raises blood pressure and puts a strain on the heart. This condition of virtually being always "on alert" will wear a person out before their time, and the inhibition of the digestive tract and the immune system further weakens them.

The adrenals require a plentiful supply of minerals and B vitamins (especially B-6) at all times, but especially in the stressful conditions in which so many of us find ourselves these days. Without these building blocks, the adrenal glands may give a spike of hormones creating a feeling of energy followed closely by extreme fatigue because they cannot keep up with the job or have run out of materials to work with. People with adrenal insufficiency will get up feeling fine in the morning but when they see their morning work, or perhaps while in the middle of a job, they will suddenly get extremely tired. Sometimes even the thought of work wears them out. For these people, any stress—whether physical, mental, emotional, financial or from whatever source—will cause the adrenal glands to either over-react and make the body either extremely tense or nervous, or else fail to respond, leaving them suddenly and extremely tired.

Nutmeg and Clove oils have corticosteroid activity. They are important to take as they support the adrenal glands and help them to heal. Clove is too hot to take by mouth but can be used on the adrenal points of the feet. Nutmeg can be "jump-started" (see Chapter 3) and used as needed. If you take Nutmeg oil, B-vitamins and minerals religiously, the adrenal insufficiency will turn itself around.

Some doctors will put patients on an adrenal glandular. There are different theories surrounding glandulars and how they work. One is that they have all the proper nutrition necessary to run the adrenals since they are chopped up and freeze-dried bovine or ovine adrenals. Another is that they will do the job of the adrenals allowing the adrenal glands to rest and heal. A third theory is that they will cause whatever is attacking the adrenal glands to attack them (the glandulars) giving the adrenal glands a rest so they can heal. I have personally known patients who had been on adrenal glandular for a number of years that never healed, although their adrenal function was improved. When they started taking Nutmeg oil by mouth every day they were able to get off the glandular and felt better than they had in years. Sometimes I will put a patient who is extremely fatigued on a glandular while feeding the adrenals the proper nutrition so that the patient can have the strength and energy needed to get up and get going. Thyromin will also help the adrenal glands if taken in the morning.

When the body has too much cortisol, even minor stress can seem overwhelming to a person. In this case we give Cortistop as directed on the bottle to our patients. Cortistop calms the body down and lowers the cortisol level. The patient begins to have more strength and energy as cortisol is lowered.

Recent research has even shown that drinking 2-3 cups of coffee per day can raise cortisol levels. Depression, anxiety, panic disorder, malnutrition and alcohol abuse can also lead to elevated cortisol levels.

Adrenal insufficiency can also cause diabetes insipidus. This is a salt-handling problem that has symptoms similar to those of diabetes mellitus. The primary symptom is thirst. It seems that you can drink constantly and still not quench your thirst. Sometimes just increasing your potassium or trace minerals helps this problem. But sometimes the problem is that the cells aren't taking up the water and it is stored somewhere else in the body instead of being utilized. Geranium oil corrects this problem by helping the cells take up water. Start by adding a drop of Geranium oil to each class of water that you drink in a day. You can eventually decrease this to a few drops a day. Once your water handling problems comes under control don't quit too soon or you will slide back to the original problem. Don't forget it takes 4 months to heal a tissue.

Recent research suggests that adrenal insufficiency may be related to or is an underlying factor in hypoglycemia. Hypoadrenia (adrenal insufficiency) is also one of the causes of chronic fatigue, discussed in Chapter 14.

On occasion I have found women who have both hypothyroidism and hypoadrenia. Upon further investigation, I usually discover that they also have a low estrogen level. After putting them on Progesterone cream and Sclaressence, I find that they get over chronic fatigue, hypothyroidism and adrenal insufficiency almost overnight.

For more information, see my book "Taming the Dragon Within" (available from Life Science Publishing).

REFERENCES

Walther, David S. Applied Kinesiology Synopsis. Systems DC. Pueblo, CO 1988

Guyton, Arthur C. Textbook of Medical Physiology. W.B. Saunders Company. Philadelphia PA. 1991

Beers, Mark H., M.D., and Robert Berkow, M.D., The Merck Manual, Merck and Co., Inc. 2005

Connelly, Dianne M. PhD, Traditional Acupuncture: The Law of Five Elements. Traditional Acupucture Institute Columbia, MD. 1994

Wertz, Dennis W., Chemistry, A Molecular Science, Prentice-Hall Inc., Upper Saddle River NJ 2002

Essential Oils Desk Reference 3rd ed., Essential Science Publishing, USA 2004

Luke J. Fluoride Deposition in the Aged Human Pineal Gland. Caries Res 2001;35:125-128

Grandjean P, Landrigan PJ. Neurobehavioural effects of developmental toxicity.The Lancet Neurology, Volume 13, Issue 3, Pages 330 - 338, March 2014 doi:10.1016/S1474-4422(13)70278-3

Thyroid. Fluoride Action Network. http://fluoridealert.org/issues/health/thyroid/

CHAPTER 16

Infertility & Sex Hormones

Infertility is becoming pandemic in the U.S. Ironically, in our abortion-plagued nation there are innumerable women who want children but can't get pregnant despite all the efforts of the medical field.

I have found in my practice that most women who cannot get pregnant have problems with their bowel and liver functions. Stagnant bowels send toxins into the uterus and a malfunctioning liver causes a hormonal imbalance. For the majority of women, doing colon and liver cleanses as outlined in Chapters 4 and 9 of this book helps correct the problem and allows them to get pregnant. It's almost miraculous.

I have assisted hundreds of my female patients in getting pregnant by teaching them the cleansing principles in this book. Most have gotten pregnant within 3-6 months of doing a colon cleanse followed by a liver cleanse. If a patient does not get pregnant within 6 months of starting these cleanses, we look at other factors such as thyroid and adrenal insufficiencies.

Of all the women I have worked with, where their husbands had viable sperm, only five did not get pregnant after doing the cleanses. These five women were all sisters and had emotional issues that they were not ready to deal with at the time.

It should be noted that none of these women smoked. Research done at a Dutch university showed that smoking more than one cigarette a day reduced pregnancy rates by 28 percent among those undergoing in-vitro fertilization, and a Canadian study demonstrated that second-hand smoke was just as harmful as active smoking. Numerous studies have shown a link between smoking and infertility, including one done in 2000 that demonstrated that smoking reduces conception rates independent of any other factor.

An article in London's Daily Times discussed the cost of infertility treatments. It said that every baby born after a single National Health Service in-vitro fertilization (IVF) treatment cost the government £13,000 (approximately $25,000). A university professor urged that the government pay for three cycles of IVF because even at a cost of up to £25,000, (approximately $48,000), a slight increase in the number of pregnancies would pay for itself in the amount of taxes each additional baby would eventually pay into the treasury. Thus IVF treatments would make a good investment, even though, according to a UK government agency, the success rate for IVF ranges only from 10.6 to 28.2 percent.

That seems a little callous to me, but I bring these things up to show the cost and unreliability of infertility treatments when the answer can be as simple as cleansing our organs. An article in the New York Times also talked about the economic ramifications of lower fertility, referring to the threat of a declining tax base resulting from the American population just barely being able to replace itself. However, the article did mention at the very end the most important reason to have children, which is pure joy.

It is tragic that so many husbands and wives wish to have children and are unable to, when the solution can be as easy as cleaning up the body's systems so that each organ can work at its optimal level.

Today's Western medicine isolates symptoms and problems without looking at the whole body. In cases of infertility the whole focus is on the reproductive system without regard to the other systems that affect it.. Medical doctors have forgotten the importance of the liver's role as a major hormone balancer. Its job is to destroy excess hormones so that there aren't too many coursing through the bloodstream, which would cause the pituitary gland not to send out more hormones. If there are too many hormones in the body it becomes unbalanced and symptomatic. For example, an excess of estrogen could lead a woman to experience hot flashes, bouts of anger or depression, weight gain, cramps or irregular cycles.

Another important factor in the body's capacity to make hormones is the liver's ability to process fatty acids. Lipozyme enzymes taken with a meal helps digest fatty acids so they can be used as hormone building blocks. Further, taking essential fatty acid supplements like flaxseed oil, evening primrose oil and fish oils helps supply the correct type of fatty acids with which to make hormones.

Other problems originate within the digestive tract itself. First, if the stomach isn't digesting proteins or if the small intestine isn't producing the proper enzymes or if essential fatty acids are not being absorbed properly, the reproductive system cannot receive the proper nourishment and the building blocks for the necessary proteins and hormones will not be available. Secondly, problems in the colon could prevent pregnancy. If the colon is sluggish, toxins from the colon can leach into the nearby tissues of the reproductive system and contaminate it so that it can't function properly.

The good news is that it usually only takes 3-6 months of colon and liver cleansing for a woman to be restored to fertility.

I saw a case once where a woman had had two children and then her period stopped for 11 years. Within 3 months of doing a colon and liver cleanse, her period started up again. A month later, she was pregnant. Unfortunately she miscarried that baby. But two months later, she became pregnant again. She carried that baby, a little girl, full term. When I last spoke to them they had had three more children and were so grateful that I had taught them the principles of colon and liver health so her body could function better.

Generally speaking, the majority of women have an excess of estrogen and a deficiency of progesterone. The body needs progesterone to get pregnant and stay pregnant. If the progesterone level in the body is too low, either the ovaries will not release their eggs or the egg when fertilized cannot attach correctly to the lining of the uterus. A natural progesterone cream such as Progessence from Young Living Essential Oils may help boost progesterone to normal levels.

Some women suffer from low estrogen and at the same time even lower progesterone. Both of these conditions may be improved by using Progessence. If the body is still low on estrogen, or was only lacking estrogen to begin with, a pregnenolone cream used either instead of progesterone or in conjunction with it may help.

Pregnenolone is the precursor to most hormones, meaning that it is the building block from which most hormones are made. The endocrine glands use the pregnenolone chemical structure and add other molecules to produce their own particular hormones.

Prenolone cream from Young Living Essential Oils is a natural pregnenolone cream, while Progessence is specifically a progesterone cream that also includes essential oils and other helpful ingredients. In my many years of assisting women with hormonal difficulties we have had the best results using creams from Young Living.

Following are some problems that arise from lack or excess of sex-related hormones and general guidelines for their treatment using Progessence, Prenolone and other natural products. These, again, are general guidelines, because everyone's body is unique.

FOR WOMEN:
Amenorrhea (No menstrual periods)
Use the new moon cycle to help you know when and how much cream to use. For example, our menstrual periods, like the moon, should be on a 28-day cycle. The hormone progesterone increases toward the 14th day just as the moon does. Then it decreases toward the 28th day. So call the new moon day 1. Wait 7 days and begin using the Progessence cream by rubbing ¼ tsp into a different part of the skin daily. Build daily until you are using ½ tsp of the cream twice daily by day 14. Then decrease until you are using ¼ tsp of cream once daily at day 28, the start of another new moon.. Stop using the cream for 7 days and begin the cycle again.

For many women with amenorrhea it takes about 3 months for the body to start having its own cycle. After you have a regular cycle use ¼ tsp cream daily.

Estrogen builds during day 1 of the cycle to day 7 with a spike of estrogen levels around day 10. Some women use estrogen products during their period. Sclaressence and Clary Sage are essential oils with estrogen-like activity. It serves some women very well to just rub 1-2 drops around their ankles 1-3 times a day. The smell of the oil alone will assist the body to start using estrogen. Some women like to take blue vervain tincture or Estro tincture from Young Living instead.

Irregular periods
Use Progessence cream as above, but count the first day of your period as day one. Start using the cream on day 7. Build as above until day 14 and decrease as above. When you get to day 28 stop the cream and wait until day 7 of your period. Sometimes you might have to wait a couple of weeks until your period starts. Do this for 3 months, then use ¼ tsp cream daily until your period is regular. Remember to stop for the first seven days of your cycle.

Period comes every 3 weeks

Use 1/4 tsp Prenolone Cream daily. Do not stop until the cycle becomes more even.

Bleeding off and on continually

Use the moon cycle as above. Stop on the new moon and wait 7 days to begin the cream. Use the cream even if you have spotting or bleeding until you get a regular cycle, then stop on day one of your cycle for seven days. Keep that usage up for 3 months, then use ¼ tsp of the cream daily.

Low Sex Drive

Add 1- 3 drops of Mister oil blend around day 15 by mouth or around your ankles. Sometimes just smelling it will do the trick. Mister boosts the male hormone testosterone, but women also need just a little bit of testosterone every month.

Excess Sex Drive

Cleanse your liver to make sure you don't have excess hormones floating in the system that the liver isn't removing. Experiment with the Progessence cream by taking up to 1 tsp of it a day to see if it will lower the sex drive. Another idea is to increase estrogen during your period and especially during day 10. Increased estrogen has been said to lower sex drive in some females while others claim that it increases their sex drive. Unfortunately, each woman is different in what is causing her excess sex drive so you will have to experiment with the hormones to see which works for you. Between day 11 and day 17 a woman should naturally have an increased sex drive as it is her body's way of signaling that it is ready to get pregnant.

Mood Swings and other symptoms

Progessence cream may also help the mood swings sometimes associated with periods. If you find your mood changing during the day, use more cream at that time. If you get a dull headache during the day then use more cream at that time. The cream may also help with painful periods, and with the cramps, heavy bleeding, water weight gain and constipation or diarrhea sometimes associated with periods. Prenolone and/or Progessence creams may also help with menopause and pre-menopausal symptoms.

Because each woman's hormone needs are different and can change day-to-day or even hour-to-hour, it is wise to test the products personally, with the help of a health professionl Also quite often there is no set recipe of how to take the products, you may have to experiment with them to see what your own body needs.

Uterus Cleansing

At times a woman might have discharges or a heavy feeling in her uterus area. I recommend cleansing the uterus if you are having these difficulties and also after every miscarriage or pregnancy. The Master Cleanse is a great way to clear the uterus. I have also had my patients use blue vervain tincture over the years, mixing 1/3 oz. of tincture with one cup warm water and drinking it all at once, once a day for three days. Other herbs I have used in a tincture combination to clean the uterus include golden root, blessed thistle, cayenne, cramp bark, false unicorn, ginger, red raspberry, squaw vine, and uva ursa.

Baby blues

Start Ultra Young+ spray and 1 tsp of essential fatty acids 3x a day about a month before the baby is due. As was noted in Chapter 10, during the last month of development a fetus requires a lot of essential fatty acids to develop its brain. If they are not available in the mother's diet the baby will pull fatty acids from where they are most readily available, which is the mother's brain. By increasing essential fatty acids such as flax seed oil or the omega-3 fish oils, mothers have experienced a decrease in post-partum depression.

A week before the baby is due, use a drop of Clary Sage around the ankles or by mouth daily. While in labor increase the Clary Sage to several drops an hour. As soon as the baby is born use 1 tsp of Progessence cream and then use ¼ tsp twice daily for several weeks. Continue using the Ultra Young + spray and taking fatty acids. You can also add B vitamins, trace minerals and calcium along with Joy and Peace and Calming oil blends. The B vitamins, minerals and calcium support the adrenal glands and the nervous systems while the essential oils give the emotions a well-deserved lift.

GENERAL:

It usually takes 3-4 months before you notice a big change in hormone production. Keep using the products for at least that long. Some people notice a change immediately while others experience more gradual improvement. But most find that their hormonal difficulties clear up within 4 months.

For more information, see my book "Taming the Dragon Within" (available from Life Science Publishing).

FOR MEN:

Male hormonal cycles

Men have hormones just as women do, and they even have hormonal cycles. These cycles just aren't as obvious or as well understood as women's. A study conducted way back in 1975 established that men have monthly cycles averaging 21 days, although there was wide variation from one man to another, and the testosterone level in these cycles varied by about 17 percent on average. There are yearly cycles as well, with the highest levels occurring in November (just in time to get ready for winter) and the lowest in April.

Men also have daily cycles. Testosterone is highest in the morning. That's when men want to get up and go, heading out to slay the dragon and bring home the bacon. Levels taper off throughout the day. One psychotherapist says that because of this daily cycle, men may be irritable, aggressive, impulsive and confident in the morning, becoming more agreeable, cooperative and passive as the day goes on. But this general pattern can be modified by events during the day. Playing sports, watching sports, or even watching or joining in anything at all that is competitive in nature brings out the maleness in men (unless he's on the losing side). On the other hand, stress is a downer, and there are a lot of stressors in today's world. Men want to take care of things that need to be put right, but there are many things that they can't personally fix – the state of the country, traffic jams, bad neighbors, poverty, money troubles, and so on. He can't slay those kinds of dragons, so subconsciously he may feel like less of a man. This may play out as aggression or depression. It helps to have a manly hobby – or at least a truck!

Then of course, there is the one-way cycle of age-related decline in testosterone. It's no secret that men lose libido as they age, and there is even a male menopause that occurs somewhere between ages 40 and 55 for many men, as testosterone levels decrease slowly but steadily after age 39.

Falling Testosterone Levels

But testosterone levels are also falling dramatically in the whole population, independent of age, indicating that there are other factors involved. The men of the 1950's had sperm counts twice as high as the men of today. Testosterone levels dropped by 17 percent just in the 20 years ending in 2007. The reason for this decline in male virility is difficult to determine. Researchers don't really know what to blame it on.

I believe that one answer, at least, may be our diets. Over the same period of time that testosterone has been declining, our foods have lost quality. I can (barely) remember when some of the first TV dinners came out, and the first meal helpers were introduced, and things have gone downhill from there. Processed foods, junk foods, genetically modified foods, additive-laden foods – they all deplete our general health, to say the least.

Actually, soy, which is an ingredient in a great many prepared foods, contains xenoestrogens. This is a threat to male health. There are many other xenoestrogens in our daily lives, including plastic bottles, cash register receipts, bisphenol A (in can linings and other places), PCB's, milk from cows treated with BST, even tap water. Few people realize that all those birth control drugs (which are xenoestrogens) women take are not filtered out by municipal water plants. These plants also add chlorine, another xenoestrogen. Glyphosate is another chemical that has become ubiquitous, to our detriment. (See Chapter 44.)

Clearly, men (and women) have to keep their eyes open if they want to avoid the dangerous chemicals that are all around us. The way men are so often portrayed as stupid bumblers on TV and denigrated as oppressors of women is also depressing to the male soul. It seems almost embarrassing to be a man sometimes.

Boosting Hormone Levels

Well, what can be done about men's hormone levels? There are plenty of supplements on the market that promise to increase testosterone, libido and performance, but I advise against hormone replacement pills. They will end up creating dependence and shutting down natural hormone production. And pharmaceutical drugs like Viagra, like most drugs, have undesirable side effects. Other supplements may be helpful, however. Many contain exotic herbs from faraway places, which we got along without just fine up until now. However, there are some things that definitely can be helpful.

Zinc is extremely important for testosterone production, along with trace minerals and vitamins in general. It is equally important for semen production and libido. Although both sexes need zinc for enzymes, immune function and general purposes throughout the body, men lose up to 5mg of zinc with every ejaculation, so they need to ingest more than women. Thus, for a healthy sex life it is crucial for men replenish their stores of zinc constantly.

Vitamin D is vital for production of sperm and for libido. Most people (men and women) don't get enough exposure to sunlight, which is the best way to get vitamin D.

We need to get plenty of healthy saturated fats, including essential fatty acids. Cholesterol, the base molecule that is made into testosterone, is a saturated fat. Conversely, we need less sugar in our diets. In general, optimizing our diets to include clean, organic foods and avoiding junk foods with all their chemicals can only help. I believe a healthy diet and a healthy lifestyle, avoiding unnatural substances, is probably the best way to maintain sexual health. Here again, "death begins in the colon."

Testosterone supplements are self-defeating. If testosterone is circulating in your bloodstream, your glands will not make it, and you will wind up dependent on supplements. Even supplementation with the hormone precursor DHEA can become self-defeating. DHEA is the most common precursor that your body uses to make sex hormones. DHEA is made in the adrenal glands, but if they are busy making cortisol so you can deal with stress, DHEA production will suffer. Thus, stress suppresses the production of testosterone. DHEA gives your body something to work with to make testosterone, which is much better than forcing testosterone on it, but in the long run it will counter-productive.

Dr. Mercola says brief, intense exercise is effective for stimulation of testosterone production. Losing weight, or more accurately, keeping the fat off, helps too, because fat stores estrogen and, of course, estrogen is the anti-testosterone. Another recommendation is to periodically "reset" your sexual health, and your general health, by fasting, which increases libido and testosterone and limits age-related testosterone decline.

Realize that sexual health, like general health, cannot be achieved instantaneously. My opinion is that artificial methods to achieve immediate results that should, instead, stem from long-term good health practices, will lead to disappointment in the end. Making sure to get enough zinc, vitamin D, exercise and so forth yield better health, including sexual health, but it's a lifestyle choice, not a momentary thing.

An occupation or hobby that makes a man feel good about himself is important to his sexual health. He needs to feel like he is worthwhile, a man who is making a difference, a man who is winning. Self esteem matters for sexual performance.

The Prostate

The prostate gland has become a trouble spot for men in recent decades. It resides near the bladder, and its main function is to make semen. Men only become aware of it if it becomes inflamed or enlarged, when it makes itself known by obstructing the ureter, which it surrounds, causing difficulties in urination. While not exactly life-threatening, this condition is annoying, inconvenient, worrisome and sometimes even painful. Prostate symptoms can stem from a prolapsed colon putting pressure on the bladder and prostate, so consider doing a colon cleanse before submitting to drugs or surgery. Patients have also had success with Protec oil blend used as an enema. It's definitely worth doing these measures before resigning yourself to drugs or surgery.

Zinc supplementation benefits both inflamed and enlarged (hypertrophic) prostate conditions, just as it does testosterone and libido. Enlarged prostate glands are always low in zinc. Of course, saw palmetto is deservedly well known as an effective remedy for prostate conditions, and is much safer than prescription drugs made from it. Other prostate-benefitting nutrients include vitamins C and D, and lycopene (found naturally in red peppers and tomatoes).

Maintaining a healthy prostate through nutrition will keep it from being a nuisance and may help prevent prostate cancer. Actually, there are always some cancerous cells throughout the body, which are defeated by a good immune system. Some men become alarmed when they are told there are cancer cells in their prostate and think they need surgery or radiation treatment, but it's a slow cancer and probably will not become dangerous. There is statistically little difference in a man's health whether he has prostate surgery or irradiation, or does neither.

Young Living Essential Oil Products for Men

Young Living makes several products for men. Prostate Health, taken daily, works very well for controlling prostate problems and helps with libido as well. It contains saw palmetto and a blend of well-chosen essential oils and other ingredients. If suffering from a hormone imbalance (lack of hormones), rub ¼ tsp of Prenelone into a different area of skin daily. Mister essential oil blend helps with libido. It can be applied to the inner cheek lining for best absorption.Also rub a drop of Mister around your ankles daily. If tests show a pituitary problem use Ultra Young+ spray.

Another blend called Goldenrod helps create what its name implies. In other words, it helps promote erections. It can be smelled or applied to acupuncture points on the ankles. These oils don't work right away like Viagra is reputed to do, and you will have to experiment yourself to see how they work for you. I do know of someone who tried Goldenrod one evening only to be woken up in the early hours of the morning with the result he had hoped for much earlier.

Case History #1

Sarah called me and said that she had heard that I was able to assist many people who were infertile to have children. I told her it was true and we arranged for her to travel several hours distance to meet with me. Because I was so confident in my pregnancy protocol I didn't pay attention to her age or what she told me of her hormonal difficulties, I just commented to her that there was no problem, that the majority of women that went on these cleanses got pregnant between 3- 6 months later, and I enthusiastically encouraged her to give it a try. Later as I was doing the paper work and reread what she had written I wondered whether I could really assist her. Sarah was a 39 year old woman who hadn't had a period in 11 years! After her second child was born her periods had stopped and she hadn't had one since nor gotten pregnant again. Within three months of doing colon cleansing followed by the Master Cleanse and the liver cleanse, she called to tell me that her periods had started again! The next month she called and said that she was pregnant. Unfortunately she miscarried that child. I encouraged her to keep cleansing and not to give up. Two months later she called to say that she was pregnant again. She carried that baby full term and delivered a beautiful, healthy girl. A year later she delivered another baby and two years later had a third baby.

Case History #2

Jessica complained to me of constant headaches. She had backaches all the time, she had severe acne, she had irritable bowel syndrome. She had severe mood swings and long bouts with depression or anger fits. Her period was irregular. It usually came every three or four months apart. When it did come she would have horrible diarrhea and be in bed for several days with migraines and abdominal cramping so bad that it would hurt from her waist to her knees.

I put her on the cleanses as outlined in this book and then told her to use the Progessence cream as outlined for amenorrhea. About six months later she called me and said, "And just why do I want to have my period every 28 days?" I asked her if she was still moody, depressed or having anger fits? I asked her if she still had irritable bowel syndrome. I asked her if she was still bleeding heavy, in bed for three days with cramping or having diarrhea problems. The answer to every question was No. That was all gone. I then said, "That is why you want your period every 28 days!" She answered, "Okay, I guess it is worth it then!"

REFERENCES

Pregnancy & Childbirth: Smoking, Being Overweight Associated With Decreased Likelihood of IVF Success, Study Says, KaiserNetwork.org Daily Reports, Apr 11, 2005 http://www.kaisernetwork.org/daily_reports/rep_index.cfm?DR_ID=29254

Passive Smoking Could Lower Chances of IVF Success, BioNews.org.uk, 27 May 2005

http://www.bionews.org.uk/new.lasso?storyid=2586

Hull, M., North K., Taylor, H., Farrow, A., Ford, W.C., et al., Delayed conception and active and passive smoking. Fertil Steril 2000; 74, 724 - 732.

Henderson, Mark, Junk Medicine: IVF Treatment, TimesOnline.co.uk, June 24, 2006, http://www.timesonline.co.uk/article/0,,8123-2238654,00.html

See FAQ, Human Fertilization and Embryology Authority, http://www.hfea.gov.uk/cps/rde/xchg/hfea

Lee, John R., M.D. and Virginia Hopkins.What Your Doctor May Not Tell You About Menopause. Warner Books. NY 2004

Lee, John R., M.D. and Virginia Hopkins.What Your Doctor May Not Tell You About

Premenopause. Warner Books. NY 1999

Northrup, Christiane, M.D. The Wisdom of Menopause. Bantam Dell. NY. 2003

Walther, David S. Applied Kinesiology Synopsis. Systems DC. Pueblo, CO 1988

Essential Oils Desk Reference 3rd ed., Essential Science Publishing USA 2004

Carlsen, E., A Giwercman, N Keiding, N Skakkebæk. 1992. Evidence for Decreasing Quality of Semen During Past 50 Years. British Medical Journal 305:609-613

Travison, TG, AB Araujo, AB O'Donnell, V Kupelian, JB McKinlay. 2007. A population-level decline in serum testosterone levels in American men. Journal of Clinical Endocrinology and Metabolism 92:196–202.

9 Body Hacks to Naturally Increase Testosterone,.http://fitness.mercola.com/sites/fitness/archive/2012/07/27/increase-testosterone-levels.aspx

Prostate Health www.medicinenet.com

Nutrition and the Prostate. http://www.doctoryourself.com/prostate.html

10 Benefits of Zinc for Men. http://health.howstuffworks.com/wellness/men/health-tips/5-benefits-of-zinc-for-men.htm

CHAPTER 17

Cleansing and Nutrition for Prospective Mothers

As I considered writing this chapter on cleansing and nutrition for prospective mothers, I decided it would be best to start in the beginning before a baby is born. I read the following account on Facebook and it was so beautiful I felt like I had to share here it.

There is a tribe in Africa called the Himba tribe, where the birth date of a child is counted not from when they were born, nor from when they are conceived but from the day that the child was a thought in its mother's mind. And when a woman decides that she will have a child, she goes off and sits under a tree, by herself, and she listens until she can hear the song of the child that wants to come. And after she's heard the song of this child, she comes back to the man who will be the child's father, and teaches it to him. And then, when they make love to physically conceive the child, some of that time they sing the song of the child, as a way to invite it.

And then, when the mother is pregnant, the mother teaches that child's song to the midwives and the old women of the village, so that when the child is born, the old women and the people around her sing the child's song to welcome it. And then, as the child grows up, the other villagers are taught the child's song. If the child falls, or hurts its knee, someone picks it up and sings its song to it. Or perhaps the child does something wonderful, or goes through the rites of puberty, then as a way of honoring this person, the people of the village sing his or her song.

In the African tribe there is one other occasion upon which the villagers sing to the child. If at any time during his or her life, the person commits a crime or aberrant social act, the individual is called to the center of the village and the people in the community form a circle around them. Then they sing their song to them.

The tribe recognizes that the correction for antisocial behavior is not punishment; it is love and the remembrance of identity. When you recognize your own song, you have no desire or need to do anything that would hurt another.

And it goes this way through their life. In marriage, the songs are sung, together. And finally, when this child is lying in bed, ready to die, all the villagers know his or her song, and they sing—for the last time—the song to that person.

You may not have grown up in an African tribe that sings your song to you at crucial life transitions, but life is always reminding you when you are in tune with yourself and when you are not. When you feel good, what you are doing matches your song, and when you feel awful, it doesn't. In the end, we shall all recognize our song and sing it well. You may feel a little warbly at the moment, but so have all the great singers. Just keep singing and you'll find your way home. The above is from The Mind Unleashed at www.themindunleashed.org.

I learned about something like this before the conception of my last child. Only instead of singing, we loved her here. We loved her with all of our hearts as we set out to conceive her. We wanted her born completely out of love not lust. What an amazing thing that did for our child. She was born such a peaceful being and she still is.

So our spiritual/emotional preparation is very important. But what about our bodies? Are they prepared to conceive and "grow" a body for a child? What can we do to prepare for that event? One important thing we can do is to cleanse.

The Importance of Cleansing Before Pregnancy

Why is it important to cleanse the body before we get pregnant? Toxins in the body can and do go through the placenta and can create problems with the baby's development. For example, they can cause neural tube defects, miscarriages, allergies, congenital defects, morning sickness (which in turn can cause malnutrition of both mother and child) and allergies in the infant. Heavy metals are dumped from the mother's body to the fetus, with the result that, according to Dr. G.F. Gordon, a specialist in metal detoxification, 600,000 babies are born with elevated mercury levels each year.

Calcium is crucial. If you don't have adequate calcium intake, the needs of the developing baby will cause the placenta to pull calcium from your bones, which will also release any toxins stored there, such as lead and glyphosate.

Avoid any and all drugs, for your baby's sake. They can and do cross the placenta. It has been found that expectant mothers who take SSRI's (selective serotonin re-uptake inhibitors) give birth to boys with 300-500 percent higher chance of autism.

Any woman who contemplates bearing a child should avoid, at all costs, genetically modified (genetically-engineered) foods, sometimes abbreviated as GE or GMO. It has been found that glyphosate, which is found throughout these plants and cannot be washed off, causes a myriad of health problems and is very difficult to remove from the body, being, as it is, a molecule not found in nature and thus without natural counter-agents. Areas of Argentina, as an example, where GMO crops were introduced 10 years ago have seen a skyrocketing increase in birth defects, miscarriages and infertility, and deadly effects are seen wherever glyphosate is used. It would be worth the effort to safeguard the child's health, and the mother's, by avoiding any and every toxin. It's never too early to start eating wisely, as glyphosate does not make its way out of the body normally, rather it accumulates. Small amounts have even been found in breast milk of mothers who were trying to avoid it. (But breastfeeding is still the best way to feed a baby.)

Another threat is xenoestrogens. Xenoestrogens are chemically made estrogen-like molecules that are widely found in soy products, plastics, cash register receipts, bisphenol-A, pesticides, herbicides etc. These compounds get in our water and in our food supply and on our skin. Our liver can't process them so it stores them in fat, especially in the breasts, hips and thighs where there are a lot of estrogen receptor sites. Having more xenoestrogens leads to a higher chance of breast and uterine cancer. And estrogen dominance is the leading cause of miscarriage. Further, in the case of a boy baby, the xenoestrogens the mother is exposed to during pregnancy have a profound limiting effect on his future testosterone levels.

In my experience and in the experience of my patients we found that if someone has had severe morning sickness in past pregnancies and then cleanses the body between pregnancies, they don't have morning sickness at all with the next pregnancy! There are many different reasons why a person is morning sick, and a toxic liver, kidney or colon is probably the major cause.

These organs along with a few others have major roles during pregnancy. It is important that they be kept clean and able to function optimally so that not only can the child develop in the best, cleanest environment but also the mother can be well and healthy during her pregnancy.

Major Organ Systems to Cleanse

I want to talk a little about the major organ systems how they affect women's hormones and also pregnancy.

First the colon: The colon's main function is to excrete wastes from the body. If it is clogged or backed up, it won't be able to get rid of these wastes. The colon has the largest blood supply in the body so as to be able to pick up nutrients and water from the chyme it receives from the upper digestive tract. If the colon is backed up, toxins will go back into the blood supply, and the liver will back up, in turn clogging the gallbladder. Secondary organs like the kidney and the skin will have to try to dispose of the wastes that can't exit via the colon, causing rashes, eczema and psoriasis, or infections or stones in the kidney. A toxic colon can leach its toxins to nearby tissues like the uterus and vagina.

Second, the liver is in charge of over 50,000 chemical functions. One of them is to balance hormones. It also aids in digestion of fats, sugars and proteins. If the liver is out of balance or toxic, the mother could experience toxemia during the last of her pregnancy. She could have gestational diabetes or severe hypoglycemia. If the liver isn't functioning optimally, she might have hormonal imbalances which in turn could cause depression, anger, bleeding, cramping, or headaches, etc.

If the liver isn't digesting fat, it begins to be coated with fat, and then other disease processes begin. The good news is that the body can heal itself. Going on a liver and a colon cleanse will clean the liver up and allow it to restore itself. But don't attempt to clean the liver until you have cleaned the colon.

How does the colon affect hormone imbalance?

First, if the colon isn't functioning right, or particularly if it is clogged, the liver backs up since there is no place for it to drain. In that case, the liver is going to have to put more toxins in storage.

Second, if the colon backs up, that invites parasites to come in. They will helpfully eat the stuff in your colon and make holes through the impacted gunk so that the colon can assimilate the minerals and vitamins and water that it needs to nourish the body. However, the parasites are also eating your needed nutrients and creating a leaky gut, and all that follows from that. As a result, the body isn't getting the nourishment it needs because the colon isn't working, plus it is feeding some little friends that have come to assist it. Now the body is going to require more food. And if you are eating more food, especially from the Standard American Diet (which is S.A.D.), you have a greater chance of consuming too many calories and too much junk that will further clog the colon.

A Remarkable Experience

When you clean the colon and the liver, the uterus will usually clean out its toxins at the same time. My friend, Jenny, found out that she had Stage 4 uterine cancer. Her oncologist told her that she was going to have to have her uterus removed and then go on chemotherapy to keep the cancer from spreading. However, she didn't want to do that. She wanted more children. She asked if there wasn't another way. Her doctor told her that if she wanted to get over cancer naturally she would have to go to another country to do it. She searched around and decided on a healing center on an island in the middle of the ocean. She went there and started their program, which was an intense colon cleansing regime. She ate a cup of bentonite clay mixed in coconut oil for her meals and that was it – no other food, no other supplements. Now, I would like to say that this isn't very balanced as far as a colon cleanse was concerned. There were no herbs or essential oils to support the body through a detox reaction. There was nothing to support either liver or kidney, two of the main elimination organs of the body. As a result, her skin broke out in horrible rashes that really itched as the toxins left the body by whatever route they could. She also did colemas in the day. (A form of high enema.) After three or four miserable months of this intense colon cleanse she had had enough and decided to quit and go home. She went straight to her oncologist and told him that she was ready to go through with the operation and chemotherapy. Upon examination, the doctor exclaimed that she was 100% healed from her cancer and that her uterus looked brand new. Now this was just from a colon cleanse! The point I am making here is that the colon is so close to the tissue of the uterus that as her colon cleansed and the toxins were removed from her body, her uterus cleansed also.

Cleanse the Uterus

I like to use Blue Vervain tincture to assist with that. Clean the uterus with 2 teaspoons of Blue Vervain tincture in a glass of water every day for three days. Generally you will feel bogginess leave the area. If you have had a miscarriage or experience heavy bleeding during pregnancy, this will assist in correcting that problem. Repeat a week later. You may experience some light brown spotting as the toxins in the uterus are removed.

After you have been cleaning the colon for a few months, you should probably worm your body to get rid of parasites and amoebas. This is simple to do by using Para Free capsules. If you have ever lived in a foreign country or a farming community, a humid state or the Midwest, you would be well advised to deworm at least once a year, or better yet, every six months. If the mother has parasites the baby will have parasites. You can see this in any animal! I know for a fact that vets come and deworm goats, cows, and horses before they give birth so that the babies will also get rid of worms before they are born!

Fixing Infertility

One of the major causes of infertility is a liver that is not functioning optimally. Because it isn't balancing the hormones correctly, a negative feedback loop begins among the pituitary, thyroid and ovaries. Probably 90 percent of the people that I work with who have infertility issues get pregnant within 6 months of cleaning their livers and colons. The other 10% have to balance their thyroids and pituitary glands. I have a consultation business for people who have trouble knowing where to start healing their body. For infertile couples, I will look at the information that I request them to send me, and I then tailor a program just for their bodies. I will teach them how to cleanse and what products and nutrition to use to get their body back into optimal health so they can conceive a baby. So if after you have cleansed the colon and the liver you still haven't gotten pregnant, go to http://doctorleanne.com to have a program tailored just for you.

Cleansing During Pregnancy

I often am asked, "What should I do if I get pregnant while I am cleansing?" I wouldn't worry about it. If you are sick or tired, continue to cleanse but if you are not and you are feeling great, you can go ahead and stop. I would like to tell you a myth that keeps going around. And that myth is that it is not safe to cleanse while pregnant. The fact is that if you are toxic the toxins will go into the baby anyway. Mothers who cleanse while pregnant have happier, more content, less colicky babies. It is especially important to do a yeast cleanse before you get pregnant and again during the last month of pregnancy. Doing so will cut down on thrush, diaper rashes, cracked nipples while nursing and baby allergies. If you are already pregnant and are very sick and feel the need to cleanse the body, I suggest you try to wait until you are 12 weeks along to be over the most important stage of the child's development. In any case, try to wait at least until after 4 weeks of gestation.

I was very ill with my first seven pregnancies. I had severe headaches and extreme fatigue and nausea. The medical/naturopath I was going during the 8th pregnancy suggested that I clean my colon . He was concerned that if I didn't, the child wouldn't get the nutrition it needed to grow. Therefore, I began to cleanse. Within a few weeks, I was no longer ill. In the past I had often been sick between months 4 and 9 with debilitating nausea. This time, it was over before I was three months pregnant. However, the best news was that when my baby was born, she was amazingly happy. She didn't have any colic. She slept easily and wasn't fussy at all. She didn't seem to have any food allergies as the previous seven children had had. What a blessing that was!

I want to say in addition, while we are on this subject of mother-baby shared illness, that when my patients bring in their nursing babies who have colic, aren't eating well and are full of gas and belly ache, I have the mother clean her colon and liver to get the toxins out of her blood and thus out of her milk, and then the baby feels better and can eat again. It works every time.

Of course, it would be better to do all this cleansing before you get pregnant as it will also help with vaginal and uterine infections, and it will help create a clean, prepared environment in which to house a growing fetus.

Adrenals are Important

Another important organ, or gland, during pregnancy is the adrenal gland. The adrenal is in charge of energy production and also makes the building blocks for hormones. Adrenal insufficiency is a chief cause of chronic fatigue and also allergies, especially asthma. If the mother has adrenal insufficiency while she is pregnant, her body will rob the baby's adrenal glands so it can run more efficiently. Thereby, the baby will be born with adrenal insufficiency and more than likely will also have allergies and asthma. Low adrenal function in the mother can also cause her to be overdue or even have a prolonged labor due to low estrogen levels during the pregnancy.

Feeding the adrenal is easy. It needs to have Super B, 1 tablespoon of cod liver, flax seed, or primrose oil, or some other form of omega oil such as Omegagize, plus trace minerals every day in order to build the hormones it makes and to create the energy hormones the body requires. The adrenal loves the essential oils of Nutmeg, Clove, Endoflex and EN-R-GEE from Young Living. Using these oils in conjunction with the adrenal balance in the Ultimate Balance book helps the adrenal gland increase its energy and improve its functions.

Estrogen Control

I want to remind you women to support your adrenal glands. When your adrenal is healthy it can make the estrogen to support you during menopause. The adrenal is the major producer of estrogen and if it is low-functioning it wants to store estrogen to draw on when a woman goes into menopause. In so doing, you might say it is saving for a rainy day, but storing estrogen causes estrogen dominance, which is an unhealthy state. It is imperative that we feed our body enough omega oils, B vitamins and trace minerals so the adrenal can carry out its functions. Reduce stress, and do emotional release techniques if necessary to assist the adrenal so it doesn't have to run on high all the time.

We need to clean out any excess estrogens in the body. Be aware that you will probably get sick as you do this, so I would strongly recommend doing the colon and liver cleanse first. While doing the Master Cleanse, you can clear excess estrogen as follows: Mix ½ tablespoon of Prenolone Cream with 5 drops of Progessence Plus. Rub this mixture all over your skin, making sure to cover your breasts, thighs, and hips with it. Use up the entire tube in a week to ten days. Repeat for 4 months. You can do this cleanse by itself, but if you are doing the Master Cleanse at the same time, it will go faster.

Colon Cleansing and the Thyroid

Most of us struggle with our thyroid issues, because our current medical system does not offer a sustainable solution apart from giving us a pill. Most medical doctors don't know about the effects of gluten on the thyroid, nor the possible benefits to the thyroid of vitamin B12 injections. And while these are good starting points, they too fall short of addressing holistically the root cause of our disease.

There are many things that affect the thyroid

The main problems are in your gut and in your liver. The health of your gut and the health of your liver are directly linked to your thyroid health. Once you fix your digestive issues, you will experience a surge of energy, weight loss, and clarity of mind, enthusiasm and clear skin. Depression and anxiety will begin to go away. You have to have a well-functioning thyroid in order to balance your hormones.

How can you know whether you have thyroid issues or whether it's really your digestive system that needs help? Well, if you are experiencing things like bloating, gas, constipation, burping, loose stool or diarrhea, or acid reflux, you have a digestive problem. In more serious cases, you might have Celiac disease or Crohn's disease, or IBS. You may crave certain foods like sweets and salt and chocolate, or starches. You feel like the day and the meal aren't complete without them. If any of this sounds close to home, it's pretty clear that your gut needs your help. How important is it to your thyroid? Let's just say it this way: you will never be able to manage your thyroid health without having a healthy gut and healthy liver.

You first need to know that 90% of thyroid conditions are autoimmune diseases. If you are suffering from hypothyroidism, you very likely have Hashimoto's disease, which is an autoimmune disease of the thyroid, even though you may not have been diagnosed with it by your doctor. What an autoimmune disease really means is that your own immune system is self-destroying your thyroid. Because of that destructive attack, the thyroid slows down, and this is the reason why you are feeling so bad.

Remember, 80 percent of the immune system lives in your gut. You will never have a healthy immune system or a healthy thyroid if you're feeling bloated, constipated, and have many different food cravings. It's key to know that the ileum (part of the small intestine) is lined with what's called the gut-associated lymphoid tissue (GALT), and is the headquarters of your whole immune system. If you are experiencing any of the digestive issues that I described, your immune system is most certainly suppressed at this point. You have to have a healthy gut to have a healthy overall immune system.

A second reason you need to have a healthy gut is to be able to properly convert the inactive T4 (thyroid hormone) to the active T3 form. The gut is one of the places this conversion takes place. If you have a healthy gut microbiome, beneficial bacteria produce intestinal sulfatase, which converts T4 to T3, but not if you are overrun with yeast and harmful bacteria.

The third reason is that our gut is responsible for the absorption of nutrients, vitamins, and minerals. Most people with thyroid conditions are deficient in many micro nutrients like vitamins D and B12, selenium, zinc and iron, just to name a few. Most people reach out for the simplest solution, which is, of course, supplements. However, when you are experiencing digestive issues, the supplements are not even getting properly absorbed by your gut. So, you are literally paying for very expensive pee and poop. Also when we absorb the vitamins and minerals properly, we feel much more satisfied with our meals much more quickly and therefore we will eat far less. Please refer to the chapters on the colon, beneficial bacteria and yeast infections for more information on the importance of gut health.

The Liver and the Thyroid

What about your liver? Why is a healthy liver is so important to thyroid health? Well, hormones and toxins are metabolized in the liver. They are excreted through our GI tract. Remember that thyroid hormones are converted into the active form in the liver. This means that your inactive T4 gets converted to the active T3 there. T3 is the hormone that gives you all your energy, clarity of mind, and metabolism; in other words, losing weight and getting the hormones to the ovaries so they can do their functions. Therefore, if your liver is sluggish, you cannot convert T4 nor a synthetic thyroid hormone like Synthroid to T3 effectively.

By cleaning out the colon, the liver and the uterus will begin to clean themselves also. By working on the liver, our hormones will begin to balance and our body will function better all around. As you can see cleansing our body has a huge effect on our hormones!

The Pituitary and the Thyroid

I would like to briefly tell you a little more about the thyroid and the pituitary gland and their importance in pregnancy. The hypothalamus and the pituitary in the brain control the normal secretion of thyroid hormones which in turn controls metabolism and reproductive hormone secretions. If these glands are not supported they may be implicated in infertility problems. The pituitary gland is important also for the signals it sends to the uterus and ovaries to begin labor, and to the breasts to produce milk. If the thyroid isn't sending signals to the ovaries, a progesterone imbalance could occur, causing the body to either miscarry or just not get pregnant. A thyroid problem can also cause problems with digestion and malnutrition. Thyroid disorders can also cause severe depression and mental illness.

The protocols to support the pituitary gland, thyroid and adrenal gland are all detailed in my book Taming the Dragon Within. It explains all about the glands involved in women's hormones and how to keep them healthy and in balance.

Nutritional Preparation for Pregnancy

Now I would like to talk about preparing our bodies for pregnancy nutritionally. There are many important nutrients that our bodies need and that the unborn baby's body needs for proper development. If you don't supply these nutrients through your diet or supplementation, the body will steal these nutrients from your bones, teeth, muscles, organs or brain!

The nutrients that I want to especially address are folic acid, iron, B vitamins, macro minerals, trace minerals, essential fatty acids, and vitamins C, D, and A.

Folic Acid is Vital

The recommended daily allowance of folic acid is 400 mcg, whether you are pregnant or not, and then 600 mcg beginning with the second trimester. This is an important nutrient to take before you get pregnant. The reason is, a lack of folic acid is a major factor in birth defects. It is the main cause of neural tube defects such as spinal bifida, cleft palate, heart disorders etc. These defects occur within the first four weeks of pregnancy, before a woman even realizes she is pregnant. So if you plan to get pregnant, make sure you buy a folic acid supplement and start taking it!

Outside of pregnancy, folic acid is important for DNA synthesis and red blood cell formation. It also, in conjunction with vitamin B-12, helps prevent macrocytic anemia, a major cause of malnourishment and chronic fatigue. These defects could also be caused by a gene mutation called MTHFR. In that case, instead of using B-12 you would need to use methyl B-12 and methyl folate. More information on MTHFR may be found in Chapter 18.

Folic acid can be found mostly in organ meats but also in certain legumes like kidney and lima beans, the cabbage family, sweet potatoes, beets and whole grains. However, this vitamin is so crucial in preventing birth defects, I strongly recommend that you buy it in a supplement and take it at least three months before becoming pregnant.

Iron

Iron is important because it is required in order for red blood cells to deliver oxygen to the cells. Without it a person can become highly anemic, exhausted and weak. Lack of iron can cause hyperactivity in children who are born to anemic mothers. It is important for making neurotransmitters and collagen. Mothers who are deficient in iron may experience weird cravings called PICA that causes them to eat odd things like ants or cleansers.

One of the strongest sources of iron is liver. Sometimes when a person is extremely tired, I put them on a diet of fresh liver, three meals a day for three days. It rapidly restores B vitamins and vitamin A as well as iron and puts them back on their feet. Other excellent sources of iron are green leafy vegetables, dandelion root and yellow dock. If you are not using poisons on your lawn, you can make your own dandelion tea by boiling three inches of root in one quart of water. Drink a quart daily. It isn't a fast remedy but it is a natural way to get iron. Some iron supplements can cause severe constipation in women or may trigger lupus symptoms. So instead of taking a supplement, eat your green leafies, especially spinach and chard. If you cook in cast iron pans, the iron from the pans will leach into your food, especially if you use tomato sauce in your cooking (because of the acidity). Tomatoes also contain iron themselves.

B Vitamins

B vitamins are some of the most important vitamins to take daily. Since they are excreted in the bowel and in the urine it is important that you have them daily. They are necessary for energy production in the body, for enzyme function, for the nervous system and neurotransmitters, for the muscles to function properly and for adrenal functions.

B vitamins:

- Support and increase the rate of metabolism
- Maintain healthy skin and muscle tone
- Enhance immune and nervous system function
- Promote cell growth and division—including that of the red blood cells that help prevent anemia.

- Reduce the risk of pancreatic cancer, one of the most lethal forms of cancer, when consumed in food, but not when ingested in vitamin tablet form.

The B vitamins are found in all whole, unprocessed foods. Processing, as with sugar and white flour, tends to significantly reduce B vitamin content. B vitamins are particularly concentrated in whole grains, green leafy vegetables, molasses, and eggs, and other good sources are potatoes, bananas, lentils, chili peppers, tempeh, beans, liver oil, liver, turkey, tuna, nutritional yeast, and brewer's yeast.

If you do not feel that you can eat enough dark green leafy vegetables in a day, I recommend you take a supplement of them. My favorite B vitamin supplement is Super B. It is a whole food supplement and does what a B vitamin should do. If you are having stress, anxiety, depression or are tired, increase your B vitamins and see how that assists you.

Vitamins C, D, and A

Vitamin C is necessary for wound healing, iron and folic acid absorption, collagen formation and strong capillary walls. Excess vitamin C in the body is excreted through the kidney. Found in citrus and tomatoes, raspberry leaf and strawberry leaf, and plentifully in Ningxia Red Juice.

Vitamin D is necessary for transport of calcium, intestinal functions, the immune system and some enzyme functions, and it fights against depression. A mere 20 minutes of sunshine will enable your body to create all it needs. Fish liver oils are another good source.

Vitamin A is used for the maintenance of certain tissues in the body including liver and eye. It's necessary for vital tooth development. Vitamin A can be found in green and yellow vegetables, sweet potatoes, yellow fruits, and butter.

Macro Minerals

The macro minerals that are of most interest are potassium, calcium, and magnesium, though there are others. Minerals are components of body tissues and fluids that work in combination with enzymes, hormones, vitamins and other transport substances. They also activate metabolic pathways. Minerals participate in nerve transmission, muscle contraction, cell permeability, tissue rigidity and structure, blood formation, acid-base balance, fluid regulation and osmolarity, protein metabolism, and energy production.

The bulk of the minerals reside in the bones; bones are mostly calcium and phosphorus. They are called macro minerals because your body needs so much of them, whereas trace minerals are needed only in small amounts. Nevertheless, trace minerals are still crucial to our bodily functions.

Doctors know that if an expectant mother has too low a calcium intake, the baby will steal calcium from the mother's bones and teeth. It is now being discovered that a mother who doesn't get enough calcium while pregnant will also have a child who will grow up needing dental and orthodontic work. The minimum requirement is 1200 mg of calcium a day for pregnant women though I have seen some recommendations for twice that amount!

Magnesium and vitamin D are necessary for the absorption of calcium. New research has surfaced that tells us we should have at least as much magnesium a day as calcium. The older recommendations were for a 2:1 calcium-magnesium ratio. Magnesium is required for proper nerve and muscle function. Many people who feel like they are stressed out a lot simply need to get more magnesium. It calms the body down, assists with the bowels and is vital for the heart to work properly.

Potassium plays a role in water balance, glucose breakdown, and carbohydrate metabolism. It is vital in nerve transmission. If you are having a lot of pins and needles feeling around the body or are extremely tired, increase your potassium and see if that assists you.

The body doesn't break down calcium carbonate without Vitamin C and B-15, but supplemental vitamin B-15 is illegal to sell in this country. Calcium carbonate also needs an acidic stomach to break down; for this reason using an antacid such as Tums to get your calcium doesn't work! The body breaks down and assimilates calcium lactate and calcium citrate much more easily than the calcium carbonate form. Sources of these minerals include apricots, sweet potatoes, meats and <u>raw</u> dairy products. Pasteurization of dairy products destroys the enzymes we need to assimilate the calcium they contain.

Trace minerals

Of all the various nutrients, trace minerals are the ones that are most often lacking in our diets. Our bodies need about 67 trace minerals, including such minerals as chromium, copper, cobalt, iodine, manganese, molybdenum, nickel, selenium, silicon, tin, vanadium and zinc. They are indispensable in enzyme functions, hormone production and sugar handling, to name a few of their uses. If you don't consume enough trace minerals while you are pregnant, the growing fetus will rob them from your adrenals and pancreas – if you have any yourself. If not, there will developmental problems.

Essential Fatty Acids

The reason that essential fatty acids (omega oils) are called essential is that the body doesn't synthesize them and they must be ingested, because the body requires them for many functions. They are necessary for hormone production, brain tissue, joint lubrication, pain relief, and the absorption of fat soluble vitamins A, D, E and K. Essential fatty acids also make HDL, which is the good cholesterol that dissolves LDL. The best source of these nutrients is the fish oils, but flax seed oil, borage oil, evening primrose oil and Omegagize from YLO are also good sources for these fatty acids. Many people's diets, and especially many expectant mothers' diets, are low in essential fatty acids, so you need to take a least a tablespoon a day to be sure of getting enough for you and the baby.

Essential Oils and Genetic Problems

I have discussed, so far, how to clean up a toxic body to get ready for pregnancy, as well as nutrition and hormone requirements. A toxic, malnourished body can cause harm to our children that ranges from birth defects to ADHD to allergies to brain damage. One of the things that I haven't addressed is genetic defects like blood disorders or immune system disorders. In that regard, I would like to relate two experiences that may be of interest to illustrate that if there is a genetic defect that runs in your family, taking Three Wise Men and Immupower in capsules from about a month before you get pregnant to the end of your third month of pregnancy may be of benefit. That will take some planning on your part to make sure your body is prepared before you get pregnant. Here are the two experiences:

One of my clients had had several children born with an immune system disorder that caused them to die shortly after birth. One child lived but had to have gamma globulin shots every month. She wanted to know what she could do to stop this problem. I told her to take Three Wise Men essential oil blend in capsules beginning at least a month before she got pregnant the next time. After she started doing that, her babies were always born healthy. We put her little girl on Immupower, a few drops in a rectal injection daily. About three months later she stopped having to have gamma globulin shots. The doctor said that something had happened. He said he could tell that her immune system was not healed but that something in the body had taken over and was providing the immune support her body needed so she didn't have to have the shots anymore.

I had another client with a blood disorder that caused her children to be bleeders. We did the same protocol as above and again the defect stopped passing on to her children. I am not attempting to diagnose your particular case nor do I guarantee you will have the same results, of course, but I offer these experiences for what they're worth, as examples of the power of essential oils.

I offer consultation packages and coaching packages to assist you with any questions, cleansing or infertility problems that you may have regarding pregnancy. I send out questionnaires to gather information on the state of your organs and your nutritional profile, and from there I can analyze what is going on in your body and come up with a program just for you. To find out more go to http://doctorleanne.com.

REFERENCES

Kilcoyne KR, et al. Fetal programming of adult Leydig cell function by androgenic effects on stem/progenitor cells. Proceedings of the National Academy of Sciences USA, doi: 10.1073/pnas.1320735111.

Case studies

I think one of the most rewarding uses of essential oils is when different techniques are combined. Here are some interesting cases from my practice.

I had a patient, Mary, present 9 months pregnant with a breech baby. We put 6 drops of Valor on each foot. I also put Valor on T-1 since that part of the spine is responsible for the parasympathic and sympathetic nervous system. As a chiropractor, I was able to find the baby's back as it lay in the womb, and I put Valor across the mother's abdomen as close to the baby's spine as I could get it. I also had the mother smell the Valor oil. I then held her feet for 10 minutes. The baby turned to the normal birthing position during the adjustment.

I have treated a lot of pregnant women. I usually had them start putting one or two drops of Clary Sage or Sclaressence essential oil blends around their ankles at the beginning of the ninth month, and also smell the oil. I had them gradually increase the amount of oil to 5 drops on the ankles daily, and in the last week of their pregnancy increase the application rate to 5 drops around the ankles 3 times a day. Three days before they were due, I had them use the Jump Start method (a drop in the mouth every minute for 10 minutes, then every 10 minutes for an hour, then once an hour the rest of the waking day). For the next day or two, while continuing to put the oil around their ankles 3 times a day, they would also take 1 drop by mouth about 5 times a day. As soon as they had any contractions, I would have them Jump Start the oils again. (We generally used Sclaressence but Clary Sage worked just as well.) When they were between 5-8 CM dilated I had them drop 15 drops in their mouths. Delivery usually occurred 15- 30 minutes later.

I never had a woman go past her due date while using this protocol. They usually delivered right on the due date. There was one woman who did go a month later than the due date the doctor gave her but it was right on the due date she had given herself at the beginning of pregnancy. One of my patients, Sarah, had had six children and had never been able to go into labor herself. She had been induced every time after being 2 weeks or more late with each delivery. She was so happy when I put her on this protocol and she went into labor by herself and delivered right on her due date.

CHAPTER 18

Children and Essential Oils

Do you have babies and children and wonder how to use essential oils on them? Perhaps you wonder how much essential oil to give a small child, or how to deliver it. Or whether cleansing might help with any of the childhood illnesses and woes, and how to do that.

Would you like to know how to take care of your children naturally for all their childhood illness such as: a stomachache, head or ear aches, burns and scrapes, asthma, flu's and colds? Would you like to know which essential oils should we always have on hand?

Essential oils are easy to use with children and babies, especially if they are pure, unadulterated essential oils. Be wary of cheaper, over-the-health-food-store-counter brands of essential oils. You may not be able to be sure whether they have been distilled with chemicals and have residues left in the oils. They may also be diluted and not work the same as top quality oils. The only brand that I recommend is Young Living, as they have been tested for their quality. Cheaper oils may burn the child's skin.

Chemical Hazards of Modern Home Life

You may not have known that DEA is a cancer causing agent that is formulated into our soaps, detergents and surfactants and, according to the booklet, "Rub a Dub Dub is there Cancer in your Tub?" is "found in over 600 home and personal care products. These products include shampoos, conditioners, bubble baths, lotions, cosmetics, soaps, and in laundry and dish washing detergents. It is just one of over 125 ingredients formulated into our home and personal care products suspected of carcinogenic activity; or, of being potentially dangerous or hazardous to our health."

Today most Americans spend 80-90% of their time inside a closed environment which could harbor over 63 of these hazardous products! We have been poisoning ourselves and our families without even knowing it. Our bodies aren't equipped to handle this many toxins! Did you know that today, one in three individuals gets cancer? This isn't to mention the rise in genetic diseases such as birth defects, asthma, lupus, ADD, and autism. Diabetes, fibromyalgia, infertility and Alzheimer's disease are on the rise. The main cause of these diseases can be traced to chemical toxicity of the (mother's) body. We absorb these chemicals through our skin and we breathe in their fumes. And what about the chemicals and hormones that are added to our food? Or the over the counter drugs and substances that we put in our bodies, including synthetic vitamins?

The Young Living Essential Lifestyle Magazine quotes a study originally posted at www.safekids.co.uk. It says: Baby lotions, eye drops, and cleaning solutions contain numerous ingredients that have officially been classified as "hazardous. " Less than a quarter of the chemicals used in toiletries and cleaning products have been subjected to a full safety investigation.

Chemicals that have been banned in other, more tightly controlled areas of the world, are still commonly used in thousands of household products in the United States. In fact the majority of commercial products sold in the U.S. contain synthetic ingredients that may be harmful, especially to small children. Most would agree that replacing chemically-based products with natural alternatives is a must, but where do you begin? Would you like to know how to get started?

Ways to Use Oils with Children and Babies

One of the most potent ways to use an essential oil is simply smelling it! It is an affective way to use oils with children. However, it is best to put one drop on your hands first, rub them together, and just pass the oil by their nose, especially if you are working with a child under two years old. NEVER use Peppermint above the navel on a child under the age of two, and I discourage using it above the feet of an infant. The fumes are too strong and can burn the eyes and shut down breathing. *If you do get any essential oil in the eyes dilute it immediately with either V-6 massage oil, olive or cooking oil or milk. Put the diluting oil straight in the eye. It will not harm the eye. Water will make the stinging worse.* A diffuser in a child's room is another way he/she can smell an oil. It goes straight to the brain through the first cranial nerve and initiates chemical changes that begin making a difference in the body.

You can also put the oils straight on the skin or rub them into the cheek lining of the mouth, but I do not recommend using any essential oil on the skin, or orally or even smelling it unless you know that it is pure and unadulterated and properly distilled. Young Living Oils uses only the highest-grade pure unadulterated essential oils.

Use Only a Little

Babies respond quickly. Don't use as much on a baby or child as you would on an older child or an adult. With a baby or child under the age of 5, think less than 1/3 of what you give an adult; 5 years to 12 years, give ½ an adult dosage and from age 12 through adulthood give an adult dosage. This pertains to essential oils and supplements.

A little goes a long way in babies and children. It makes huge difference quickly in a baby. Some oils you may need to dilute as children have sensitive skin. You can put an oil neat or undiluted on a child's skin but remember babies and children have sensitive skin and be ready to dilute with V-6 or vegetable oil at the first sign of discomfort.

Vitaflex Method

Usually you can put an oil straight on the foot and Vita-flex it in. The Vitaflex method is actually one of the most effective ways to use essential oils on a child. Babies and children respond very quickly to this method. Vitaflex is a technique where you apply the oil on the foot to a specific acupressure point, then rub your finger over this point, rolling from the pad of the finger to your nail. Make sure you have short nails so you won't scratch the child.

The Essential Oil Desk reference and my book Ultimate Balance both have charts that show where the Vita-flex points are on the feet. If you have a child with bowel problems it is easy to put DiGize on the feet and Vita-flex it on the Large Intestine points, This helps the child tremendously with having bowel movements.

If a child does get too much of any oil in the mouth, give him or her a tablespoon of olive oil or coconut oil as soon as you can to dilute it. This will quickly stop the reaction that they may be having. Babies may react in different ways if they have too much oil. They may cry, they may flush either in the face or on the skin. They may hyperventilate or foam at the mouth. Note, I have never seen those last two reactions in children, but I have seen it in animals. We helped the reaction by giving the pet olive oil in its mouth.

In the Bath

Baths are also another wonderful way to assist your baby or child with essential oils. Lavender, for example, helps relax the baby or child. Always combine the oil with Epsom salts before adding it to the water so that the oil won't float on the top and possibly burn the skin if the oil is all in one spot. This is especially important with a hot oil such as Peace and Calming or Oregano or Peppermint. If using Peppermint in a bath, make sure to add the Epsom salt/oil mix after you turn off the water so the steam or mist won't pick it up and spread it through the room causing tearing of eyes. Mix the Epsom salts around to dissolve them. With a baby or small child use only ¼ cup or less of Epsom salts in the tub.

Rectal and Enema Applications

Rectal injections and enemas are great ways to get an essential oil into a baby or small child. I prefer to mix the essential oil 5 drops of essential oil to 1 -2 tablespoons (15-30ml) of cold water. When mixed with cold water, the water rapidly drives the essential oil into the tissues of the colon, decreasing the chances of stinging or burning in the tissues.

Enemas are great for fevers and congestion. Doing an enema pulls the mucus from the body. Peppermint brings down the fever and helps to release mucus. An enema hydrates the body. You can use a Peppermint enema on a baby as long as the infant doesn't smell the fumes. For lung issues in a child see the "Cold sheet treatment" in Appendix E. Don't forget to decrease the amounts given in the instructions to better suit a baby or child.

Some Useful Oils for Children

Let's first talk about different oils and how you can use them. Then we will take a different tack and discuss some common problems and how to use essential oils and cleansing techniques to assist the child in healing.

Lavender – This is the first oil I choose when working with children and babies. It is a mild, gentle oil and is great for bruises, burns, swellings, skin abrasions, ear infections, teething, inflammation, relaxation, sleeping problems, cankers.... You can put it on straight; usually you don't need to dilute it even for babies.

My son James, at age 18, was having his wisdom teeth come in and his gums hurt. Since I had used Lavender on my babies when they were teething, I figured it would likewise soothe his gums. Within a few minutes of applying Lavender, he had relieve of his swollen gums and tooth pain. A few years later, another teenager in the family had wisdom tooth pain. She chose Clove oil and had similar results.

Di-Gize™ - For children I would chose Di-gize for gas or stomach upset. Rub on the stomach or Vitaflex the stomach point on the foot, or put it on your index finger and rub it in in their cheek lining. (Be careful of touching the tongue. Kids may not like the taste)

From a mother of several children: Taylor does not like Peppermint so I use fennel when she has a stomachache. (Fennel is the main oil in Di-gize) A few days ago we ate out at a restaurant and she was doubled over in pain from gas, so I put a little fennel with olive oil on her lower stomach and within a few minutes she was sleeping very peaceful.

Melrose™ - Here is an oil that I would never be without. It is excellent for any skin problems especially skin abrasions, sores, burns, rashes, infections and insect bites.

I love Melrose. I make sure I am never out of it. A number of years back, my 9-month old baby burned her finger in a gas heater pilot light that she somehow reached. The tip was burned black. I put a drop of Peppermint on the tip to stop the pain then alternated Melrose and Lavender on it several times a day. I put a bandage on it to keep the oil away from the baby's face. Within a week, the burn was gone and the finger looked like new.

Raven™ - Raven is a perfect oil blend to use for chest congestion or other lung issues. Raven has several types of eucalyptus in it that help break up congestion. Another ingredient is Ravensara, which is specific for lung tissue. However, it doesn't work on asthma, because asthma is a muscular problem in the bronchial tubes, not a congestive problem. Marjoram and Citrus oils work better for asthma.

My friend, Rebecca, tells this story about the essential oil blend Raven:

"When my youngest was 6, she developed a nasty croupy cough. She woke up after a late afternoon or early evening nap gray and struggling to breathe. I rubbed Raven all over her feet, back and chest and within minutes she began to cough and gag. She then vomited mucus. She vomited so much mucus she filled a large, family sized salad bowl. Immediately her color came back. Instead of the former pale, bluish-grey color, her skin was now pink and back to normal. I had my baby back and she was ready to get out of bed, eat and play."

R.C.™ - R.C. stands for respiratory congestion. It is similar to Raven but is intended more for upper respiratory issues. It can be used for a runny nose, sinus problems, and insect bites. RC seems to activate the body's histamine response while it keeps the itching down by also acting like an antihistamine. This action is what makes it great for insect bites and hives. You can use RC on the sinus points of the feet. The fumes may be too strong to place it on the child's face.

Gentle Baby -This is comforting, soothing, relaxing and beneficial for reducing stress. Just the name alone tells you its purpose. It is particularly soothing to dry, chapped skin and diaper rash. It is wonderful to put into the bathwater along with a drop or two of Lavender to relax a cold or infant. When done before bedtime it will assist an upset child to sleep better without bad dreams.

Lemon - Lemon increases microcirculation and lymphatic function. It is stimulating, invigorating, and promotes a deep sense of well being. It has been shown to lift moods and act like an antidepressant.

Peppermint - This is a wonderful oil to use on acute pain, like when a child slams their finger in a door. It stops the pain instantly; it is a powerful pain blocker. It also has anti-inflammatory and anti-spasmodic properties making it excellent for stomach pain, gas, and headaches on a child more than two years old. The menthol in Peppermint oil helps open the sinuses. Rub some Peppermint oil on your hands then do a quick pass by the child's nose, repeating until the nasal and sinus pathways open.

Purification – Purification is perfect for disinfecting and cleansing cuts, scrapes, bug bites, and splinters and other little hurts. It works well in a diffuser to cleanse and disinfect the air to neutralize mildew and disagreeable odors. This will assist in keeping down airborne germs and mold that might contribute to allergies.

Panaway - Reduces pain and inflammation, increases circulation, and accelerates healing. Relieves swelling and discomfort from sprains, muscle spasms and cramps, bumps and bruises.

Thieves - This is a blend of highly antiviral, antiseptic, antibacterial, anti-infectious essential oils. It is fantastic to keep colds, and the flu at bay. You can rub it on tick bites to bring down any inflammation. Many mothers in rural areas have used it on a tick bite that shows the first signs of Lyme disease. Their children never developed Lyme's. A number of Thieves fans have been eager to share their stories:

Mrs. Kauffman puts a drop of Thieves in her children's apple juice or orange juice every morning. They haven't missed school for illness since she began doing this.

Terrie Look from Vermont shares the following: A couple of years ago when my children were in 1st and 4th grades in their very small school of 125 students in northern Vermont. The school had to postpone their Christmas concert until after Christmas because over 40% of the school (children and employees, alike), were home sick for over a week with a deeply nasty flu! My children did not get sick, and did not miss any days of school that winter. I had been diffusing Thieves and Purification into our house, and applying minute amounts of Thieves neat on the soles of their feet (one of the quickest and most effect ways to disperse essential oils into the body) and in a small amount of veg carrier oil to the base of their spines (where viruses like to hang out) each night and morning. Thieves is one of our all-time favorite oil-friends!

Billi Tribe from Australia adds: Our family which includes my 3 daughters, husbands and 8 grandchildren under 7 years old uses Thieves and RC at the first sign of a cough or running nose, it's also great for sinus problems. We apply RC on the chest and back and across the cheeks for sinus and Thieves under the feet on the children. The symptoms normally stay mild and we are back to good health within 24 to 48 hours. The adults put a drop or 2 of Thieves on their tongue at the 1st sign of viruses. It's also a great idea to put Thieves on the soles of the feet of school aged children to help prevent them from picking up viruses etc at school.

Dina Klein from North Dakota says: I have faithfully been using Thieves (since January) to ward off the cold and flu's of this season. At the end of March I was exposed to some severe chest colds and sinus infections. My day had also been sick for over a month when his turned ugly. Whenever I felt a tickle in my throat I would put about 3 drops of Thieves oil in my mouth and by morning the tickle would be gone. This even worked with a very sore (knife feeling) throat that came on one night. Thieves is amazing.

Lena Wolfe from Alberta, Canada advises: Thieves oil, when diffused, is extremely powerful. Last winter, I started diffusing Thieves oil as soon as I had my new diffuser, from Young Living, of course. Which was in December of 2006. Our immunity towards colds, flu-bugs and all the "fine" viruses floating in the air during the winter, was dramatically improved by doing so. We also drink NingXia Red, which is also very beneficial for sooo many things that it would take too long to list.

Virginia Graham from Texas comments: We just love the Thieves oil blend. For colds and flu, go for Thieves. Sore throat? A drop of Thieves in water, gargle and swallow. Or try Thieves spray - one spray does the trick. Thieves lozenges are great, too, especially for the little ones. Thieves cleaner is "my" cleaner for everything, from cabinets and high chairs, to all bathroom fixtures, doorknobs and dishes. Thieves toothpaste is a must, and safe for the whole family.

Cheryl Meier from Wyoming states: I have been operating a child care for the past thirty-five years. Of late it has been tough with the number of viruses the children have arrived with. This past year, we started diffusing Thieves oil in the child care, and using Ravintsara and Raven directly on the children as they surfaced with runny noses or coughs, with written permission from the parents. From the time we started applying the essentials oils and diffusing we have experienced not one lost day to child care due to illness. One little toddler who had been on a nebulizer since birth was able to exist without it after been introduced to the essential oils and being taken off dairy. I can not possibly share the total improvement we have enjoyed in health with all of the small children we care for.

Valor - Valor balances energy to instill courage, confidence and self-esteem. It helps the body self-correct its balance and alignment. Use it nightly on the feet and spine to balance the nervous system.

Little 8-year old Sarah B. had nightmares every night. After putting Valor on her feet and up her spine and especially on the base of her neck, she stopped having nightmares and began to sleep soundly.

I would like to talk about different ways to cleanse a baby or child to help rid them of certain ailments. The following conditions can be helped greatly with cleansing.

Allergies

First off, how do babies get food allergies? Why is this happening? Wouldn't you think that they would be clean when they're born? These are questions a parent might ask.

The answer is, when a baby is born with allergies, it means the mother was either extremely toxic while the baby was in utero, or was not taking the nutrition necessary to support her adrenal glands while carrying the baby, or didn't have good gut health to digest her foods. A less likely possibility could be that she has the MTHFR mutation and now so does the child.

How do you help a baby to get over allergies? Can you even do a colon cleanse or liver cleanse on your baby? And why would you have to do so?

The first thing to do is to support the child's adrenal glands. This can be done by Vita-Flexing Nutmeg oil on the adrenal points on the feet. Using Mighty-Vites spray will also assist in giving the child some B-vitamins that strengthen the adrenal glands. I think that giving a child ½ teaspoon (2.5 ml) of olive oil, flax seed oil, or cod-liver oil with one drop of Juva Cleanse essential oil blend will not only assist in cleaning out the liver but will also help in building up the adrenal gland to where it should be. Or you can rub Nutmeg oil on the baby's feet and mid-back area at night or several times during the day. If you are nursing the baby, double the amount of Super B you are taking. Rub olive oil or cod liver oil on the baby's skin so the oil will soak through the skin and into the body. You can also give the baby 1/2 tsp of olive oil per day in the mouth.

Stool Health

If within the first week after birth the baby's stool doesn't start turning yellow but remains green, this is evidence that the liver needs cleaned out. It is easy, as the following experience will show.

Just recently, I had a client whose baby presented with severe allergies. This two-month-old baby still had green stools. I had the mother VitaFlex the baby's feet with JuvaCleanse and put Juva Flex under the right rib cage. I also had her give the baby 1/2 teaspoon of olive oil by mouth. That cleans out the liver and helps it start to digest better. It also helps change the stool to yellow. The stool cleared up in a couple of days and the allergies disappeared. But why would a tiny baby need to clean its liver, you ask. Because its mother was toxic during her pregnancy and the toxins passed through the placenta.

If the baby is exhibiting a lot of constipation the first step is to get them adjusted by a chiropractor who knows babies. Sometimes when babies are born, especially if they had too fast a birth, a traumatic birth or forceps on the head, they need to be adjusted to get the "kinks" out of their spine and head and pelvis; many times it takes a lot of adjusting to get them straightened out. That will also assist the colon in working better. If the colon is still not right, let them drink sweet potato water, the water that you boiled sweet potatoes in. If you think of it as an herbal tea and not a food, your head can handle it better! It cleans out the colon and assists it in functioning better.

A pediatrician once told me that it is common for a baby not to have a bowel movement for 10 days. I would like to say that it may be common but it isn't normal! Starting a baby out right with bowel and liver function right after they are born will assist it in being healthy without allergies or other digestive issues.

A Compromised Immune System

A mother asked the following question regarding a condition that I have seen in many children. "I have a 3-year old that is allergic to everything, and I mean EVERYTHING–eggs, cow's milk, almonds, cockroaches, mold, trees and grass. She is not allergic to peanuts though (thank goodness). She has been on a constant prescription of Zantac and Zyrtec since she was about six months old. We have restricted her diet to avoid the food allergens, but even so if she misses one dose of the prescriptions she breaks out in TERRIBLE hives. Her lips swell huge, her eyes swell shut, and her ears are double their normal size. I believe this all started with her vaccinations, but obviously cannot say that for sure, I just know that after each round of shots the allergies got worse and worse so I stopped them. Any help/advice is greatly appreciated. Thanks!"

This was my answer: "I believe the problems your toddler is suffering come from a compromised immune system, stemming from a lack of beneficial gut bacteria. Often this originates with the mother not having healthy gut bacteria when carrying the baby, and the problem continues if the baby is not breast-fed, because the infant is slower to acquire these bacteria if not breast-fed. Gut bacteria play a critical role in developing our immune system. Next, the vaccinations we are almost forced to give little babies further damages the immune system, which has not had the opportunity to develop properly in infancy anyway.

"Zantac is used to reduce stomach acidity. I can't see how that would be a good idea. Reducing stomach acid hampers the digestion of proteins, and undigested proteins combined with an unhealthy colon leads directly to allergies. Zyrtec is an anti-histamine, so evidently it is being used to reduce allergic symptoms. Young Living products that could more safely be substituted include R.C.and NingXia Red.

"NingXia Red is rich in vitamin C and acts as a wonderful anti-histamine. It supports the immune system of the body.

"What we need to do first is to reduce the inflammation in the gut and then rebuild the micro-environment in the colon. Health is based upon this foundation. (Hippocrates said all disease begins in the colon.) If your child indeed has compromised gut flora as I suspect, grains are probably irritating the bowel lining. I suggest you eliminate grains and grain products from the diet temporarily. Grains are not bad for us, but the way they are processed into store products of all kinds is not healthful, and it will be hard to fix the gut if it continues to be irritated. Sugar of all kinds should also be avoided; they feed yeast and bad bacteria in the gut. Cut out grocery-store milk and milk products, but if you can find a great organic yogurt, it would be very helpful.

"A probiotic supplement such as Life 5 from Young Living is crucial. One capsule a day is probably plenty for a small child. It would be easier to put it into applesauce or water or something than to get that big capsule down a child's throat. In addition, any fermented foods you can get the child to eat, such as sauerkraut (or yogurt), for example, will help re-establish the proper colon bacteria. You can ferment vegetables yourself (there are instructions online) to give her, if she will eat them. Nevertheless, even non-fermented vegetables will help. I suggest you include sweet potatoes, bananas, legumes and nuts in her diet. These will provide fermentable fiber for the good bacteria to work on to help the colon heal. Sweet potatoes in particular are great for gut health. If she is allergic to almonds, it may be just the kind you have available in your store. Organic almonds might not cause a reaction (just a suggestion). Soaking the almonds for several days in liquid whey also assists them to be more digestible. Meat is okay. You might be surprised to learn that butter is very important for gut health. Let her eat all the butter she wants. Use coconut oil in place of all other oils and fats.

"Finally, I recommend you give your child a rectal injection of Lavender or Idaho Balsam Fir essential oils every day for a week. Put about 4 drops of either oil into a teaspoon of coconut oil and use a rectal syringe to inject it. You may want to warm up the coconut oil a little so it is in liquid form when you add the essential oils then let it cool down before injecting it into the rectum.

"Once the inflammation has decreased in the colon and the gut flora re-established, her allergies should begin to go away. In addition, she should be able to eat and digest more foods.

"Doing all of these things, should assist the immune system to work better against the food allergies and histamines. The gut will begin to work better and the enzymes should improve to digest the food."

Preventing Allergic Reactions

Here is an experience with children and essential oils graciously shared by Pat Tukey, from Washington:

"I have several friends with children who have allergies/asthma that come and visit my farm. Normally after 15 minutes in my barn, and around my animals, they come out with swollen eyes, stuffy noses, red faces, and going to "Mom" for Benadryl, or inhalers, or what have you.

"I got rather frustrated so made a rule that if these children wanted to be in my barn, they had to use two oils before entering! First I had them put Lavender on the palm of one hand, rub their hands together, and then wipe their hands on their faces, necks, and arms, and anything not covered. I had them do the same with Peppermint, but only had them inhale this from cupped hands over their noses, but not wiping it on themselves.

"Now these kids can spend hours in the barn with no ill effects - no runny noses, no swollen eyes, etc. I was amazed and delighted because now they can spend time with the animals which they love."

Milk Allergy

I have seen small children with milk allergies, especially if they are being formula fed, but even breast-fed babies!

In the case of a breast-fed baby, I will have the mother do a liver and a colon cleanse first while still nursing to clean out her own toxins so the baby won't be getting so many toxins in the milk. This is often the case with colic; the mother's milk is toxic and is upsetting the baby's digestive system. Mothers, I would recommend cleansing your body. Do not be afraid that the baby will get your toxins through your milk if you cleanse. IT ALREADY IS! If you cleanse with The Cleansing Trio from Young Living, it will bind the toxins and remove them from your body. Grapefruit oil and Juva Cleanse Oil really help with removing toxins from the blood.

Some babies are born without the enzymes necessary to digest milk, or some other food. (This is common in children with autism and in that case could be a DNA issue.) If milk allergy is a problem, remove the baby from cow's milk immediately. Milk seems to be the first food allergy that shows up because it is the first potentially allergenic food they eat. Cow's milk has proteins that are very hard to digest. It is not like the proteins in human breast milk. Goat's milk is closer to breast milk. Some Amish milk their horses because it is even closer yet.

The first sign that a child is not digesting milk is a shiny rash on the cheeks, and sometimes also on the forehead and on the head itself. Sometimes it gets crusty like milk would if you didn't wash it off. If you don't take the baby off milk, the allergy doesn't go away, it just changes. A baby doesn't grow out of a milk allergy, the symptoms merely change as the baby grows. The mucus membrane gets affected. Runny noses start. Ear infections begin. Bronchitis sets in. Then if you still don't take them off milk the body starts making a drug similar to opium. Now you have a child who either will have ADHD or ADD. Next, other food allergies start taking over. Now you and the baby have real problems.

If you are nursing a baby and it seems to be reacting to your milk, try taking cow's milk out of your diet. If that doesn't help, add enzymes to your diet to assist you in digesting the proteins you are eating. In the section on eczema I discuss further steps to clear up allergic reactions.

Autism Spectrum Disorders

ADHD, Autism, Asperger's syndrome, OCD, Oppositional Defiant Disorder plus others such as Rhett's syndrome and Angelman's syndrome can all be found on the Autism Spectrum Disorder continuum. They can be helped with essential oils.

There has been a lot of debate as to whether vaccinations are the cause of this disorder. It is a rather hot debate. I have my own opinion. One of the things I have found of most interest over the years is the work by the Pfeiffer Clinic in Naperville, Illinois. They found that people with this disorder seem to be missing a gene that makes the protein L-Methionine which in turn makes an enzyme that handles metals in the body. Hence, a cascade of events begins to happen. The metals mess with the trace minerals in the body causing the body to not be able to digest gluten or casein. (Casein is a milk protein.) Without this enzyme and in combination with heavy metals, the body makes opiate-like compounds out of the casein and gluten giving you a child on drugs. The first order of cleansing, then, is to take these children off gluten and dairy. Some people see a tremendous difference in their children within months of taking them off these foods. The website http://www.gfcfdiet.com/ has all manner of gluten-free, casein-free (GFCF) recipes to help people who have this problem.

MTHFR Gene Mutation

Pfeiffer Laboratory worked over the years to find out how to solve this problem of the missing gene. Meanwhile, Defeat Autism Now (D.A.N.) doctors found through their research that methyl B-12 shots and magnesium chloride really helped these children. The breakthrough came when the actual mutated gene was discovered. It is called "methylenetetrahydrofolate reductase (NAD(P)H)" and nicknamed Monday Thursday Friday (MTHFR) for short. Some of the conditions a person who with a MTHFR mutation (and there are many different variations) may have include severe chronic depression, ADHD, autism, Asperger's, lupus, celiac disease, food allergies, skin sensitivity, sensitivity to the sun, inability to lose weight, or hyper-histaminia. It has further been noted that people with this gene mutation cannot process pharmaceutical drugs, so drugs don't work for them, which is a common complaint in lupus patients. A sufferer may have many symptoms or just a few, and person with more than one mutation of this gene would have worse symptoms than if they had only one. Autoimmune conditions may be more common in those with MTHFR mutations. Women who have MTHFR are also at risk of miscarriage, and there may be an association with spina bifida in their children. Therefore, checking others in the family for this gene, and treating with folinic/5-MTHF and Methyl B-12 may be helpful in minimizing many chronic diseases.

Cleansing and Children

So what can we do about this condition besides adopting the GFCF diet? A cascade of ill health is happening that must be addressed. Dysbiosis, inflammation and yeast are the primary ones. We need to first repair the gut. (See Chapters 4, 5 and 7) Another early intervention "must" is to rid the child of metals. Children can cleanse for metals. In the chapter on metal cleansing I have a great cleanse using Young Living oils and products to assist in pulling heavy metals out of the tissues, binding them and moving them out of the body.

Note that metal cleansing is not easy on the body. It makes symptoms worse while the metals are mobilized. But being able to defeat them with many of our Young Living products really helps. The best method is to mobilize the metals one day, bind them that day and the next, and then rest a day or more before you mobilize them again. This cleanse is made for adults so make sure that you only use a third or less of the oils and products on your child to make it easier on them. If your child cannot swallow a pill you can open the capsule and combine it with something that they child will eat. For example we used to mix ICP and other powders in refried beans or a whipped topping for our son and he would eat that without a problem.

L-Methionine makes a huge difference in being able to handle metals. The symptoms seem to go away quickly. If the child has a mutated MTHFR gene I suggest you keep him on L-Methionine forever. Ask your DAN doctor to assist you in finding out if your child needs this. We started putting my profoundly autistic son on Methyl B-12 shots and within a few weeks he began to imitate us! That was an incredible development, because he had never been able to connect at all before that. Unfortunately, I can't tell you the end of his story as he got sick with a bad flu along with the rest of the family and, having always had a weak constitution, died a few weeks later. I would like to have seen what else might have happened with this treatment.

Oppositional Defiant Disorder

Oppositional Defiant Disorder is on the Autism Spectrum Disorder. I think that Surrender oil blend is about perfect for that one. I worked on a child who had this disorder as well as Obsessive Compulsive Disorder. As long as I adjusted her head with Highest Potential essential oil blend she would be fine. I had to adjust her monthly. I told the mom to keep the Surrender and Highest Potential on her head. As long as we did that she didn't have any problem with her disorders. After of a few months with oils and adjusting she was fine and no longer had the disorders.

OCD is a spleen issue. Do the energy work for it outlined in Ultimate Balance. ODD can stem from a wheat allergy. I know that as long as my daughter didn't eat wheat she didn't have that issue. (She has Asperger's). She is now an adult and beginning to try the Methionine to see if that will allow her to eat wheat and calm her emotions down. Wheat allergy can come from small intestine issues such as SIBO or from a yeast infection.

Before you start on a metal or liver cleanse be sure that you first give the child a colon cleanse. If your child is less than one year old and you think he or she needs a cleanse, give him or her, instead, things are very healing to the gut. As you continue to read through this section more colon and liver cleansing ideas will come forth.

A Formula that Helped Autism

My son had profound autism and mild cerebral palsy. When he was 8 I asked Gary Young what I could do for him. He gave me the formula below to use in a Raindrop massage on him three times a day, along with a rectal injection twice a day. After a few weeks of this he got up and took his first steps. That was an exciting day! He had never walked or crawled before.

Here is the formula:
20 drops Frankincense
20 drops Idaho Balsam Fir
20 drops Myrrh
20 drops Conyza (Flea Bane)
5 drops Peppermint
3 drops of Valor on each foot.

As was noted in Chapter 7, one doctor stated that he had seen more than 1000 cases of autism reversed through anti-fungal treatment, or yeast cleansing.

ADD/ADHD

ADHD and ADD are increasingly common among children, especially boys. According to a government study, the incidence increased 22 percent between 2003 and 2010, although it is quite possible it is over-diagnosed for the purpose of giving children drugs to keep them under control. Two-thirds of children diagnosed with ADHD are on medication. Part of the problem may be that children don't adapt well to being cooped up, as shown by the fact that spending more time in nature is a viable part of treatment. But much of the blame may be placed on poor diets, including junk foods containing too much sugar, glyphosate and additives, not enough healthy fats, and lack of support for beneficial flora in the gut. Gluten sensitivity and chemicals in the child's environment may also be at fault.

I once saw a video of Dr. Terry Friedman taking the brainwaves of a child with ADD. ADD is the version of ADHD where the child is not necessarily hyperactive, but cannot concentrate. They may sit quietly and just stare into space. He put the probes on the child's head and we saw that the child had Theta brain wave activity. You can think of Alpha brain waves as the waves you would see if you are just relaxed or even in a meditative state. Beta brain waves occur when a person is thinking, learning, and very aware of their surroundings. Delta brain waves are the sleep waves, and Theta waves are the deep sleep waves. You would really need to shake a person hard to get any response if they are in Theta sleep.

To return to the story, here was this child, awake and yet his brain was in Theta wave deep sleep. Dr. Friedman put some Brain Power essential oil blend on a cotton ball and gently put it up the child's nose. Instantly the brain waves on the monitor switched to Beta Waves, and the child became alert.

I have used this treatment on many children who couldn't concentrate in school. We put Clarity, Present Time or Brain Power on terra cotta necklaces. Some of the boys didn't want to use the necklaces so we put one of the oils on a small wad of cotton and used a bandage to hold it in place. These children had huge changes in their ability to focus on their schoolwork.

One boy, Noah, went from the bottom of his class to the top of his class in grades using this method. His mother also said that after coming home from school, instead of going to lounge on the couch or his bed, he went straight to his chores and got them done.

CHAPTER 19

Perils of Modern Times: Diabetes, Obesity, Allergies

Type II Diabetes

Diabetes has become a burgeoning problem in the United States in recent years. Diabetes is the opposite of hypoglycemia, which was discussed in Chapter 14, in that blood sugar levels are too high—due to insufficient insulin—rather than too low. Elevated blood sugar is a very dangerous condition that often leads to heart attack, high blood pressure, or stroke because the red blood cells will tend to clump together creating a thick, sluggish blood that could cause a blockage in a small artery, with a resultant lack of oxygen in a critical area of the heart or brain. Diabetes also gives rise to many other disease states in the body, including neuropathies, kidney failure and loss of eyesight.

Though sometimes treated the same way by medical doctors, Type I and Type II diabetes are two completely different disease states. Type I occurs because of a genetic defect or a virus in the pancreas that destroys the cells in the Islets of Langerhans that produce the hormone insulin.

All the cells of the body (except for brain and liver cells) require insulin in order to take in glucose, which is their fuel source. Insulin also is necessary for protein synthesis. A person with Type I diabetes, the inability to produce sufficient insulin, is usually diagnosed at a very early age, and must take insulin for life. A person with Type II diabetes, on the other hand, is usually age 30 or older when diagnosed. This person is typically overweight and sedentary and may consume alcohol excessively, all of which are major risk factors for becoming a Type II diabetic.

A very great tragedy in the U.S. is the number of people becoming diabetic at younger and younger ages, chiefly as a result of excess sugar consumption and lack of exercise. Have you ever seen an overweight child or teenager waddling around with a large soft drink in hand? That is a poor soul on the road to diabetes.

Unlike type I diabetes, Diabetes II doesn't stem from a problem in the pancreas, but rather from a problem with the insulin receptor sites on the cell membranes. The pancreas produces plenty of insulin, but because of the excessive amount of glucose to which the insulin receptor sites are constantly exposed, and other issues, they become resistant to insulin and therefore can't pass glucose into the cells. The insulin receptor sites also become fewer in number.

According to the report of the Second World Congress on the Insulin Resistance Syndrome, currently 65 percent of Americans are overweight, with 24 percent having the insulin resistance syndrome. But for people born in 2000, the lifetime risk for developing diabetes is up to 33 percent for men and 39 percent for women. The trend is in the wrong direction!

Medical doctors generally suggest that someone with Type II diabetes watch their diet and exercise more to keep the disease under control. This is good advice. In research studies, a 5 percent reduction in weight led to a 74 percent reduction in diabetes and more than 4 hours of exercise a week led to an 80 percent reduction in diabetes. (By the way, lifestyle change was shown to be much more effective than medication.) But too often people would rather do anything than change their lifestyle. The obliging doctor prescribes some pills in an attempt to keep the blood sugar down, but the condition usually progresses to requiring insulin shots. Even with this regime, though, I have quite often seen patients whose blood sugar is still way too high.

A key element for treating Type II diabetes is to clean up and rejuvenate the insulin receptor sites. I have seen reversals of diabetes II by people who do a colon cleanse, a Master Cleanse and then a liver cleanse. The Master Cleanse does a fantastic job of cleaning insulin receptor sites.

Chapter 6 explains how to do the Master Cleanse, but if you have Type II diabetes you should change the recipe of the lemonade in the Master Cleanse to use molasses instead of maple syrup, because molasses doesn't enter the blood stream as rapidly and cause the blood sugar to spike. Purification oil blend from Young Living taken by mouth also cleans up cell receptor sites.

Another problem that occurs in Diabetes II is that the liver does not handle sugars well. Cleaning out the liver allows it to function at its optimal level, so it is important to do a liver cleanse as well as the Master Cleanse. I also recommend drinking NingXia Red juice blend as a general tonic.. This is especially useful when the liver is not at its best, or during a liver cleanse, because the juice helps the liver with its function of regulating the blood sugar levels. I take ¼ cup at a time. If in 15 minutes the problem is not improving, I take another ¼ cup. Alternatively, you can take Coriander essential oil sublingually (a drop under the tongue) if blood sugar is too high, one drop a minute until it comes down.

An additional way to help deal with elevated blood sugar levels is to take an enzyme between meals that digests sugars. I have my patients who are cleansing take Essentialzymes-4, because it is formulated to digest carbohydrates and sugars, as well as fats and proteins.

In addition to reversing their diabetes, people who follow this regime will also begin to lose weight and feel better energetically. This, in turn, leads them to begin exercising. Enlightened patients will also begin to take better care of themselves by changing to a healthier diet that includes fresh fruits and vegetables, whole unprocessed grains, fewer saturated fats and less protein. They stop eating empty-calorie foodstuffs like potato chips or cakes, donuts, cookies and other pastries or sweets. It's worth the effort to be free of diabetes!

Obesity

Obesity is one of the leading health issues in the U.S. today. The topic is constantly in the news. I have heard some scientists suggest it is simply species genetics; that our genes are simply evolving to create bigger and heavier people. Although we dance around the subject, it is an open secret that our 'widespread' obesity stems largely from unhealthy practices, not least of which is our Standard American Diet (SAD) with its heavily processed foods. Sadly, the SAD has spread to other "advanced" countries too. At the International Congress on Obesity held in September 2006, experts said an obesity pandemic threatens to overwhelm health systems around the world with illnesses such as diabetes and heart disease. "We are not dealing with a scientific or medical problem. We're dealing with an enormous economic problem that, it is already accepted, is going to overwhelm every medical system in the world," said Dr. Philip James, the British chairman of the International Obesity Task Force. He said the costs were immeasurable on a global scale but estimated it at billions of dollars annually in English-speaking countries. Estrogen and growth hormones in milk doubtless contribute to obesity, and fluoride is a causative factor in hypothyroidism, which has as one of its symptoms weight gain. Attention has been focused recently on the fats used in food preparation in fast-food restaurants. A scientific reiew of Harvard School of Public Health concluded that drinking one can of soda pop per day could cause 15 pounds of weight gain in a year.

In reality there are many factors involved in weight gain or loss. A good friend of mine, Dr. Susan Schultz, coined the acronym SHED to highlight these factors, which are Stress, Hormones, Exercise and Diet. Each of these factors must be considered in our fight against obesity. If these factors are out of balance a person will gain weight and will not be able to lose it no matter what they do.

STRESS:

If stress is high a person tends to overeat the wrong kinds of food. Yet, good diet and exercise are ways to lower stress!

HORMONES:

Hormonal imbalance, either estrogen dominance or hypothyroidism, will lead to weight gain. Depressed adrenal function makes it difficult to even want to get up and exercise.

EXERCISE:

Sitting around watching TV all day or even working a desk job has made a generation of lethargic individuals who don't get enough exercise. Yet walking just half an hour a day not only burns calories so a person can lose weight, but also lowers stress, one of the other factors in weight loss. As a side benefit, walking improves PMS problems.

DIET:

I have said a lot about our SAD diet and its effects on our health in this book. My diet recommendations are included below.

So what do you do if you are overweight? To begin with, cleansing the body as outlined in this book does wonders for weight loss in several ways. Toxins do have weight and are mostly stored in fat cells. As you cleanse the body those fat cells that encase the toxins are purged. I know from personal experience that when the lining of my bowel came out, I lost 25 pounds all at once. Some patients have remarked that as they cleanse the kidney and the body, they have lost 10-35 pounds of water weight over the course of a few days.

As you do your cleansing, balance the hormones, work on your stress levels and start a good exercise program. Begin with stretching and weight lifting to build muscle, and then walk every day for at least half an hour. Walking uses all the muscles in the body, thus keeping them toned and burning calories. Walking has the added benefit of activating the lymph system, allowing wastes and toxins to clear from the body.

Most importantly, change your diet. Eat food as close to its raw, natural state as you can, avoiding the ills that come with processed carbohydrates, unnatural fats and innumerable food additives. The more raw vegetables, fruits, nuts and grains you eat in place of processed foods, the healthier you will be. It's almost impossible to know what additives have been added to our food along the way, thus my recommendation to eat avoid processed foods as much as you can. For example, on August 18, 2006, the FDA approved a "cocktail" of six viruses to be sprayed on ready-to-eat meat and poultry products (think lunch meat and hot dogs), to combat a certain rarely-encountered bacteria, at the request of a biotechnology company. What the consequences of our consuming these viruses will be down the road, I have no idea. I doubt anyone can keep track of all the additives the FDA has approved of, or yet will, so I recommend you eat simply.

Grains can be made into sprouts and eaten in salads, giving much higher vitamin value than simple grain kernels. Lowering your consumption of meat (you actually need only 2 ounces a day of protein) is a significant step in creating a more alkaline and thus healthier body. By all means rid your diet of the empty calories found in things like cakes, cookies and other desserts.

If you must drink milk, drink raw organic milk that hasn't had its enzymes destroyed by pasteurization, its healthful fats beaten into strange molecules through homogenization, and isn't full of hormones.

Learn to eat only when you are hungry and to stop when you are full. Drink more water. If you think you are hungry, have a drink of water first and see if you weren't really thirsty instead of hungry. Cut out caffeinated drinks, soda drinks, and alcohol.

Add essential fatty acids to your diet. The body's appetite will often not be satisfied until it has enough of the fatty acids it is lacking. By taking a teaspoon of flaxseed oil, fish oil or olive oil before a meal you will find that you stop overeating because the body has satiated itself on what it was looking for in the first place.

If you have done all of the above—cleansing, de-stressing, balancing hormones, exercising and changing your diet habits—you will find that you don't have to go on a stringent calorie-counting diet to release weight. It will just automatically come off as a by-product of your better life style.

Allergies

Allergies are caused by the body's inability to digest proteins properly. Because it isn't digesting proteins well it has too many foreign proteins floating around in the blood stream. Then when it comes in contact with another foreign protein such as grass pollen or fruit tree pollen it sends histamines to attack the protein and you get an allergic response such as watery eyes.

The best long-term solution to allergies is to do a colon and liver cleanse. In my practice, the vast majority of people who had allergies, no matter whether it was animal, plant, airborne, chemical or otherwise in origin, really benefited from colon and liver cleansing. In most cases cleansing was sufficient to clear their allergies.

Yeast or parasites can also cause allergies. A person with an overgrowth of yeast in the colon typically has allergies along with it. However, I have found that doing a yeast cleanse or parasite cleanse alone doesn't quite clear up allergies because the yeast and the parasites usually cause damage to the colon walls and the colon has to heal. Colon cleansing repairs the colon because the herbs in the cleanse help build back the damaged tissues.

The adrenal glands can also contribute to allergy problems. In this case it usually manifests as asthma. Supporting the adrenals takes care of most asthma conditions.

For the most part, allergies that erupt on the skin like hives, rashes, etc., stem from a colon or liver malfunction. Colon or liver problems can also leave the body susceptible to airborne allergies that cause hay fever or runny noses and sinusitis. Food allergies fit in this category as well. Smells or chemical intolerances are also usually a liver problem. It is a great idea to clear the systems every year through seasonal cleanses to keep the body toxin-free and to ensure that the body continues to digest its foods and nutrients properly, thus preventing allergies.

I first became interested in natural healing because of the numerous allergies I had, and now I can say I don't have any! If I occasionally break out in hay fever, I know that it is a sign I need to do a colon and liver cleanse or that I have stressed myself out and need to support my adrenals.

I have mentioned dealing with allergies in several chapters of this book, but I would like to gather everything together here for the sake of convenience.

First and foremost, as I have reiterated throughout this book, do a colon and a liver cleanse. Meanwhile here is a list of measures you can take for relief of specific symptoms:

- **Runny nose**: Use a drop of RC oil blend on the upper gum every minute for 10 minutes or until the nose dries up, or use a few drops of a mild saline solution in each nostril several times a day.

- **Sinusitis**: Use RC on the upper gum as directed above. Put it on the cheeks and on the bridge of the nose at the beginning of the eyebrow being careful not to get it in or near the eyes. Breathe in Peppermint oil as it will open the sinus cavities. Breathe in the steam from cooking onions, garlic, parsley and cabbage all together.

- **Hives:** Take 1- 5 Juva Tone capsules. Apply RC, Purification, Melrose, or Lavender directly on the hives. Hives will respond in seconds to the correct oil, so experiment with different oils until they do respond. NingXia Red juice blend is an excellent anthistimine as it is full of vitamin C. Drink an ounce every 15 minutes until symptoms decline. Onions are also a great antihistamine. Fry them up and eat them!

- **Skin Rashes:** Take Juva Tone capsules as above. An enema with either Peppermint or Purification oils (5 drops in 2-3 cups of water) will help clear the lower colon of toxins that might be causing the rash. Adding JuvaCleanse oil blend (about 5 drops) or lemon juice to the enema will help clear toxins from the liver. Many times this will immediately bring down an acute rash. More chronic rashes like eczema or psoriasis will clear up after several months of cleansing.

- **Asthma:** Citrus oils have been scientifically shown to stop an asthma attack. Just breathing the oil in will often stop asthma within a few minutes. Support the adrenals as mentioned in this book.

Some allergies in babies are caused by a reaction to milk. This usually shows up at first as a red glistening rash on the cheeks that can eventually spread over the entire head. Next it progresses to a constant runny nose, then frequent ear infections, then asthma or chronic bronchitis. Taking the child off milk products clears this problem up.

There have been a number of deaths from peanut allergy in the last few years. We didn't see this at all when I was a child. I have to wonder whether there is some new chemical being put on the peanut crop that is really the cause of the problem rather than the peanut itself. Nevertheless, peanuts are sometime a serious problem so be cautious of them if your child has a lot of allergies, especially a yeast problem. Most people who have yeast infections cannot tolerate peanuts. Dr. William Crook and other nutritionists maintain that peanuts are prone to mold and that in itself can contribute to allergies and more yeast problems, whatever other allergy factors may enter in.

Allergies wear down the immune system, so while you are cleansing the body make sure you build the immune system by cleaning out the lymph glands, using such products as ImmuPower or Immunetune to help build lymphocytes and white blood cells. I recommend you also support the bone marrow with Rehemogen, since the marrow is the source of new blood cells.

Case History

Rachel had such severe allergies that she had to leave her house every Saturday morning so her children could deep clean it with commercial cleaners, then air it out before she could come home. If the grass got too long and went to seed she had to wear a mask over her nose and mouth so she could breathe. She had terrible hay fever in both the fall and the spring. She had severe food allergies and couldn't tolerate many foods. She was constantly using decongestants and antihistamines for chronic sinusitis. She was allergic to animals of all kinds, dust, birds, pollens, chemicals, and the list goes on. She had asthma and chronic bronchitis. She couldn't walk down the soap aisle in the supermarket without sneezing and coughing and becoming nauseous. She had a bowel movement every 10 days and thought that was normal. She also suffered from skin rashes, hives and vaginal yeast infections.

We followed the protocols outlined in this book. I had her first do a colon cleanse, and then a kidney cleanse, followed by the Master Cleanse and finally a liver cleanse. Within 4 months she free from all allergies except for wheat, milk and apples. She continued cleansing for several more months and was completely relieved of all of her allergy symptoms. She faithfully ate only natural foods for about 3 years before letting white flour products, sugar and milk creep back into her diet and stopped doing yearly cleansings. About 7 years after the first cleanse began to get severe hay fever again as well as asthma attacks. She remembered the cleansing protocols and started to cleanse again. By the next fall her hay fever was gone, as was the asthma.

Beginning with that cleanse she decided to follow my recommendation of cleansing each organ according to its season for just a few weeks each season. She has remained allergy-free for the past three years.

REFERENCES

Walther, David S., Alpplied Kinesiology Synnosis, Systems DC, Pueblo CO 1988

Guyton, Arthur C., Textbook of Medical Physiology, WB Saunders Company, Philadelphia PA 1991

Beers MD, Mark H., and Berkow MD, Robert, The Merck Manual, Merck & Co. 2005

Bloomgarden MD,Zachary T., Second World Congress on the Insulin Resistance Syndrome, Diabetes Care 28:2073 Aug 2005

Ford ES, Giles WH, Dietz WH: Prevalence of the metabolic syndrome among US adults: findings from the third National Health and Nutrition Examination Survey. JAMA 287:356–359, 2002

Ludwig DS, Peterson KE, Gortmaker SL. Relation between consumption of sugar-sweetened drinks and childhood obesity: a prospective, observational analysis. Lancet 2001; 357:505-8.

Schulze MB, Manson JE, Ludwig DS, et al. Sugar-sweetened beverages, weight gain, and incidence of type 2 diabetes in young and middle-aged women. JAMA 2004; 292:927-34.

Vasanti S Malik, Matthias B Schulze, and Frank B Hu, Intake of sugar-sweetened beverages and weight gain: a systematic review Am J Clin Nutr 2006 84: 274-288

Health Experts: Obesity pandemic looms, http://news.yahoo.com/s/ap/20060903/ap_on_he_me/obesity_conference

Healthy Weight, Harvard School of Public Health http://www.hsph.harvard.edu/nutritionsource/healthy_weight.html

Pereira MA, Kartashov AI, Ebbeling CB, Van Horn L, Slattery ML, Jacobs DR Jr, Ludwig DS. Fast-food habits, weight gain, and insulin resistance (the CARDIA study): 15-year prospective analysis. Lancet. 2005 Jan 1-7;365(9453):36-42.

FDA CFSAN/Office of Food Additive Safety. FDA Approval of Listeria-specific Bacteriophage Preparation on Ready-to-Eat (RTE) Meat and Poultry Products http://www.cfsan.fda.gov/%7Edms/opabacqa.html

Essential Oils Desk Reference, Essential Science Publishing USA 2004

Randolph, Theron G., MD. and Ralph W. Moss Ph.D., An Alternative Approach to Allergies. Harper &Row. New York , NY.1989

Rochlitz, Steven. Allergies and Candida With the Physicist's Rapid Solution. Human Ecology Balancing Sciences, Inc. Setauket N.Y. 1989

CHAPTER 20

Building Blocks of Better Health

W hile cleansing the body or, at the very least, soon after the cleaning, it is important to make sure that you are also getting the kind of nutrition that builds the body. I like to call this nutrition "builders." Cleansers go through the body and clean out the toxins, allowing the body to be clean so it can heal itself. Builders give the building blocks to the body so it can rebuild and strengthen the tissues.

Builders include vitamins, minerals, essential fatty acids, essential sugars and proteins. Notice I didn't say chemicals! The aforementioned nutrients are the proper chemicals of the body. Vitamins and minerals and sugars are used in chemical reactions, and proteins are the catalysts of those chemical reactions. Fats and proteins make the hormones that trigger the enzymes to make the chemical reaction. Sugars create the cell-to-cell communication in the body. Vitamin and minerals make the energy reaction in the body and it is the vitamins and minerals that are the neurotransmitters for the brain! The nervous system runs on calcium and B vitamins, including choline! Reading through a good book on clinical nutrition, you will be amazed at what these nutrients do!

And where do these nutrients come from? Ideally, from the food that we eat! But if you aren't digesting your foods or are eating food devoid of nutrition, you will need supplementation. It is often necessary to use supplements at the beginning of the healing process as the body needs more of certain nutrients then. For example, essential fatty acids (EFA's), more frequently called omega oils, are some of the nutrients that most systems of the body need in order to function. If you are truly healthy you only need a teaspoonful of an omega oil per meal. But to repair tissue, you need a quarter cup of essential fatty acids a day for 4 months, or until the tissues of the body heal. As I said, most tissues need EFA's, so if you have a lot of healing to do it may take more than 4 months to heal all the tissues of your body.

In the health questionnaires that I give people to ascertain the health of their organ systems, I list 15 systems. I have listed next to these systems some of the most important nutrients that each system needs to repair itself. Notice how many are similar:

Stomach . . . . Omega oils, trace minerals, B vitamins
SM Intestine . . . . Omega oils, trace minerals, B vitamins, Macro minerals
Lrg intestine . . . . Omega oils, trace minerals, B vitamins, Macro minerals
Gall Bladder . . . . Omega oils, trace minerals
Liver . . . . Omega oils, trace minerals
Spleen/Pancreas . . . . . Omega oils, trace Minerals
Adrenal . . . . Omega oils, trace minerals, B vitamins, Macro minerals
Pituitary . . . . Omega oils, trace minerals,
Thyroid . . . . Omega oils, trace minerals, Iodine
Heart . . . . Omega oils, trace minerals,
Lungs . . . . Omega oils, trace minerals, B vitamins, A and D
Kidney . . . . Omega oils, trace minerals, B vitamins, beans, nutmeg
Immune System . . . . . Omega oils, trace minerals, B vitamins
Nervous system . . . . . Omega oils, trace minerals, B vitamins, Macro minerals
Reproductive system . Omega oils, trace minerals, B vitamins

It's clear that most of the organ systems and glands need trace minerals, omega oils and B vitamins to either build tissues or to carry out their daily functions.

Essential fatty acids:

Essential fatty acids, also popularly called omega oils, are not made by the body so it is "essential" that we get them in the foods that we eat. Mostly we need to be aware of our omega-3 intake; we generally get enough of the other omega oils.

Not all fats are good. Avoid the fats that present a high workload for the liver and gall bladder. These are margarines, processed vegetable oils, partially hydrogenated fats/trans fats, deep fried foods, foods that are not fresh and contain rancid fats, and processed meats. In those with a dysfunctional liver, I recommend avoiding all processed animal milks and substituting instead oat, rice, almond or <u>organic</u> soy milks. (Avoid soy milks made from genetically engineered soybeans).

Eat the "good fats" which contain essential fatty acids in their natural unprocessed form. These are found in cold-pressed vegetable and seed oils, avocados, fish (especially oily fish such as salmon, tuna, sardines, herring, sablefish, flounder, trout, bass and mackerel), shrimp, prawns and crayfish, raw fresh nuts, raw fresh seeds such as flax seeds (linseeds), sunflower seeds, safflower seeds, sesame seeds, hemp seeds, alfalfa seeds, pumpkin seeds and legumes (beans, peas and lentils). Flax seeds and others can be ground freshly every day (in a regular coffee grinder or food processor) and added to cereals, smoothies, fruit salads and vegetables. Spirulina, evening primrose oil, black currant seed oil, borage oil and lecithin also contain healthy oils to help the liver. Do not use margarine on your breads and crackers. Replace it with fresh butter, tahini, humus, pesto, tomato paste or relish, freshly minced garlic with cold-pressed oil (chilli or other natural spices can be added if enjoyed), nut-spreads, fresh avocado, cold pressed olive oil or honey. The good fats are essential to build healthy cell membranes around the liver cells. As we get older we need to "oil" our bodies and not "grease" our bodies.

Essential Sugars:

Essential sugars are an important part of a balanced diet when used appropriately. Research over the last 25 years has actually confirmed that not only are sugars good for us, some are essential (just as some amino acids and fatty acids are essential in our diet).

Though it is better to get these sugars through the foods that we eat, the body does have a secondary mechanism within the chemistry functions of the body that makes these sugars, though at great expense to the energy stores of the body.

Here is a list of the essential sugars that our body needs to use for either cell-to-cell communications, support or energy production.

1. **Mannose (polysaccharide)**

   Properties: Anti-bacterial, anti-fungal, anti-viral. Reduces inflammation.

2. **Fucose (simple sugar)**

   Properties: Anti-viral. Supports long-term memory. Guards against lung diseases. Fights allergies. The abnormal metabolism of this saccharide is associated with cystic fibrosis, diabetes, cancer, and herpes - more fucose helps to alleviate these conditions.

3. **Galactose**

   Properties: Improves the speedy healing of injuries. Improves memory. Improves the absorption of good calcium

4. **Glucose (simple sugar)**

   Properties: Fast energy source. Too much or too little can be problematic. Glucose metabolic disturbances are associated with depression, manic behavior, anorexia, and bulimia. Glucose is the body's preferred energy source for the brain and all other tissues but is best derived from more complex sugars and carbohydrates.

5. **N-Acetylgalactosamine (polysaccharide)**

   Properties: Inhibits the spread of tumors. Heart disease causes a low-level of this saccharide.

6. **N-Acetylglucosamine (polysaccharide)**

   Properties: Immune system modulator. Anti-viral. Anti-inflammatory. Repairs cartilage. Repairs the mucosal-lining that is damaged by Crohn's disease, ulcerative colitis, and interstitial cystitis. Enhances learning.

7. **N-Acetylneurominic Acid (polysaccharide)**

   Properties: Anti-bacterial, anti-viral. Enhances learning and brain development. Abundantly found in breast milk.

8. **Xylose (simple sugar)**

   Properties: Anti-bacterial, anti-fungal. Helps prevent cancer of the digestive system.

There are more sugars than just these eight (just like there are more amino acids than the 8 or 9 essential amino acids). The list of food and herb sources of essential sugars (listed above) is by no means complete. Generally, if you eat superfoods (wolfberries, goji berries, bee pollen, marine phytoplankton, aloe vera, etc.), medicinal mushrooms (reishi, cordyceps, maitake, Lion's mane, etc.), and seaweeds (especially kelp powder, nori, dulse, and sea lettuce) you will get all the essential sugars into your diet naturally. A well balanced diet (not a SAD diet) should provide the nutrition you need. You will have to go beyond just grabbing whatever is convenient, though.

In general, berries are the best class of fruits as they contain glucose and a larger amount of healthful medium- and long-chain polysaccharides than most other fruit types. Try different types of medicinal mushrooms. Start with Reishi. Experiment and discover which ones work best in your body. I personally enjoy Reishi.

Please note that the Ningxia Red Juice from Young Living has at least 6 of these essential sugars in it. The others can be found in Sulfurzyme and BLM.

9. **Amino Acids (Proteins):**
Consume a diverse range of proteins from grains, raw nuts, seeds, legumes, eggs, seafood, free range chicken and fresh, grass fed, red meats. If you do not want to eat red meat or poultry, there are many other sources of protein. Strict vegetarians can get adequate protein, however, you may need to take supplements of vitamin B-12, iron, taurine and carnitine to avoid poor metabolism and fatigue, and zinc supplementation is often required. To obtain first class protein, strict vegetarians need to combine 3 of the following 4 food classes at within 18 hours of each other so they can combine to become a "whole protein" - grains, nuts, seeds and legumes, otherwise valuable essential amino acids may be deficient. If your body is lacking amino acids you will be fatigued and you may suffer with mood changes, reduced cognitive function, hypoglycaemia, poor immune and liver function and hair loss. I have met many strict vegans who felt unwell because they were lacking amino acids, iron and vitamin B 12, and after supplementing with these nutrients and modifying their diets they quickly regained excellent health.

10. Vitamins and Minerals

Their sources and where they are found:

Vitamins	Sources	Function
A	Cod liver oil, sweet potatoes, carrots, leafy vegetables, and fortified foods such as breakfast cereals.	Needed for good eyesight and normal functioning of the immune system.
B-1 (Thiamin)	Enriched, fortified, or whole-grain products such as bread, pasta, and cereals.	Helps the body process carbohydrates and some protein.
B-2 (Riboflavin)	Milk, breads, fortified cereals, almonds, asparagus, dark meat chicken, and cooked beef.	Used in many body processes, such as converting food into energy. It also participates in the metabolism of many drugs and helps in the production of red blood cells.
B-3 (Niacin)	Poultry, fish, meat, whole grains, and fortified cereals.	Aids in digestion and converting food into energy. Also used by the body to help make cholesterol.
B-6	Fortified cereals, fortified soy-based meat substitutes, baked potatoes with skin, bananas, light-meat chicken and turkey, eggs, and spinach.	Vital for a healthy nervous system. Helps the body break down proteins. Helps the body break down stored sugar.
B-12	Beef, clams, mussels, crabs, salmon, poultry, soybeans, and fortified foods.	Needed for creating red blood cells and general cell division.
C (Ascorbic acid)	Citrus fruits, red berries, tomatoes, potatoes, broccoli, cauliflower, brussels sprouts, red and green bell peppers, cabbage, and spinach.	Helps promote a healthy immune system and is required to help make collagen, which holds cells together. It is also required for making chemical messengers in the brain.
D	Fortified milk, cheese, and cereals; egg yolks; salmon; and sunlight.	Needed to process calcium and maintain bone health.Important other effects on all cells of the body.
E	Leafy green vegetables, almonds, hazelnuts, and vegetable oils like sunflower, canola, and soybean.	Functions as an antioxidant.
Folate (Folic acid)	Fortified cereals and grain products; lima, lentil, and garbanzo beans; and dark leafy vegetables.	Vital for cell development, prevents birth defects, promotes heart health, and helps red blood cells form.
K	Leafy green vegetables like parsley, chard, and kale; olive, canola, and soybean oils; and broccoli.	Helps clot blood and maintains bone health.

Minerals	Sources	Function
Calcium	Dairy products, broccoli, dark leafy greens like spinach and rhubarb, and fortified products, such as orange juice, soy milk, and tofu.	Helps build and maintain strong bones and teeth. Helps muscles function. Involved in cell communication and signaling.
Chromium	Some cereals, beef, turkey, fish, beer, broccoli, and grape juice.	Helps maintain normal blood sugar (glucose) levels.
Copper	Organ meats, seafood, cashews, sunflower seeds, wheat bran cereals, whole grain products, and cocoa products.	Aids in metabolism of iron and red cell formation. Helps in the production of energy for cells.
Iodine	Iodized salt, certain seafoods, kelp, and seaweed.	Works to make thyroid hormones.
Iron	Leafy green vegetables, beans, shellfish, red meat, eggs, poultry, soy foods, and some fortified foods.	Needed to transport oxygen to all parts of the body via the red blood cells.
Magnesium	Whole grain products, leafy green vegetables, almonds, Brazil nuts, soybeans, halibut, peanuts, hazelnuts, lima beans, black-eyed peas, avocados, bananas, kiwifruit, and shrimp.	Helps muscles and nerves function properly, steadies heart rhythm, maintains bone strength, and helps the body create energy and make proteins.
Manganese	Pecans, almonds, legumes, green and black tea, whole grains, and pineapple juice.	Involved in bone formation and wound healing, metabolism of proteins, cholesterol, and carbohydrates. It is also an antioxidant.
Molybdenum	Legumes, grain products, and nuts.	Plays a role in processing proteins and other substances.
Phosphorus	Dairy products, beef, chicken, halibut, salmon, eggs, and whole wheat breads.	Helps cells function normally and help the body make energy. Helps red blood cells deliver oxygen. Important in the formation of bone.
Potassium	Broccoli, potatoes (with the skins on), prune juice, orange juice, leafy green vegetables, bananas, raisins, and tomatoes.	Aids in nervous system and muscle function. Also helps maintain a healthy balance of water in the blood and body tissues.
Selenium	Organ meats, shrimp, crabs, salmon, halibut, and Brazil nuts.	Helps protect cells from damage and regulates thyroid hormone action and other processes.
Zinc	Red meat, fortified cereals, oysters, almonds, peanuts, chickpeas, soy foods, and dairy products.	Vital to many internal processes and supports immune function, reproduction, and the nervous system.

CHAPTER 21

A Few Words About Detoxification Reactions

My husband once said to me, "Cleansing seems so counter-intuitive. Here you are feeling worse today than yesterday." One would think that if you ate something and woke up sick the next day, that you wouldn't want to eat that ever again. (I do have a friend who won't cleanse for that very reason.) But what I know is that I want that stuff out of my body. I really don't want the metals and toxins messing with my enzymes, spleen, adrenal, brain, or causing cancer anymore. I want lupus to go away and leave me alone. I want to have energy and life again so I will go the distance.

When it comes to the various disease states, some can have a hard detox reaction. Some of the "hard" cleanses are bacterial infections, yeast or candida detox and metal detoxing. I have tried to warn you throughout the book, which ones might be a little tougher than others and for all cleanses I warn to clear the major pathways first with colon and liver cleansing.

Adolf Jarisch and Karl Herxheimer published descriptions of the detox reaction in 1895 and again in 1902. This reaction is sometimes called "Herxing" or "Herx" or "the JHR". Not everyone will go through it. It depends on the severity of the problem being corrected and the type of treatment being applied. Herxing occurs when dead or dying bacteria, or toxins such as yeast die-off or metals, release in large amounts into the blood stream. This creates a major and sudden inflammatory state. In my opinion, this happens when the patient's immune system is already low and taxed. It seems that when the white blood cell captures the bacteria they both die, causing increased pain and inflammation and more WBC's to be called to the scene. And the bones start to ache as the marrow goes into overdrive to make more white blood cells. Do not worry, it is the body's response to an invasion of sorts.

According to the Chronic Illness Recovery website, "The most common symptoms reported include increased fatigue, joint or muscle pain, skin rashes, photosensitivity, irritability, paresthesia, dizziness, sleep disturbances, asthenia, muscle cramps, night sweats, hypertension, hypotension, headaches (especially migraines) and swollen glands. Also reported are heavy perspiration, metallic taste in mouth, chills, nausea, bloating, constipation or diarrhea, low grade fever, heart palpitations, tachycardia, facial palsy, tinnitus, mental confusion, uncoordinated movement, pruritus, bone pain, flu-like syndrome, conjunctivitis and throat swelling".

I have experienced such reactions and have added into my protocols ways to make it easier for people to get through them. The following are some additional treatments you can use to assist you in detoxing while cleansing.

One of my favorite ways to assist my body with detox reactions is to bathe in Epsom salts and Clove oil. I mix 5-15 drops of Clove oil with 1-2 cups of Epsom Salts and fill the tub with water as hot as I can stand. Hot water also stops pain reactions as it overcomes the nerve for pain since heat and pain run on the same nerve pathway to the brain. The Clove and Epsom salt mix draws toxins out of the skin. About 20 minutes into the soak you may discover black "gunk" being released from the skin, and it may itch. If you do see that, scrub it off with a loofa sponge. When it has released, the aches and pains seem to leave the body. You can also add 1 cup of apple cider vinegar or a cup of baking soda. Adding 10 drops of Ginger or Peppermint essential oils to the tub will assist the body to start to sweat. This sweating will assist in drawing out the toxins in the body. Drinking warm Peppermint of Ginger tea will also assist the body in building a fever and sweating. The purpose of the fever is to allow the immune system in making new WBC to fight the inflammation that is going on. Have glass or two of water handy to drink. If you start getting faint, cool down the water in the tub and drink the water you have brought. Ask someone to assist you in getting out of the bathtub so you will not faint if you are dizzy or lightheaded. This feeling means that you have pulled too many minerals from your body. Replace them with by drinking NingXia Red with a little Mineral Essence. Rehydrate the body by drinking more water and then lay down to rest.

Another way to pull toxins from the body is to use a foot ionic bath such as a B.E.E.F.E or EB305 machine.

While cleansing, it is important to drink distilled water, which will assist in picking up toxins. It also binds with minerals so it is important to replenish macro and micro minerals while cleansing. Losing magnesium and calcium during a cleanse, for example, can lead to tight muscles, jangled nerves and added stress to the body as the adrenal gland starts wearing down.

I always make sure to take more Comfortone and ICP during detox reactions. A good thought to cheer you is gratitude that you are killing off the pathogens making you ill!

I also jump start either Juva Cleanse or Purificaion oil by mouth. As a reminder, to make a big change quickly, such as for low adrenal function, stomach flu, or sinus problems, or for detox reactions, you can "jump-start" the organ by using essential oils as follows: Take one drop of essential oil by mouth every minute for 10 minutes, then one drop by mouth every 10 minutes for an hour, and then one drop by mouth every waking hour for the rest of the day or until you feel better. If you rub the drop in the buccal mucosa (inner cheek lining) of the mouth, it doesn't leave such a bitter or tangy taste as it would on the tongue, and it is absorbed more readily. You can always use a chaser like a piece of bread to rid yourself of the taste of the oil if you don't like it.

NOTE: Not all essential oils are for oral use. If you are going to use one orally, it is extremely important that you use only therapeutic grade essential oils that have been organically grown and steam-distilled. This will insure that you don't ingest chemical fertilizers, herbicides or pesticides used in growing the plants, or chemical solvents or other toxins used in processing the oils. Further, not even all therapeutic-grade oils are intended for internal use. Check the label!

Taking Detoxzyme between meals also assists the body in chewing up the toxins being released.

Please note that when you are mobilizing heavy metals, the detox reaction can be quite intense. Blood purifiers such as red clover and yellow dock can help, as also do Lemon oil or juice enemas. In addition, using L-Methionine will assist in digesting metals quickly but it might also remove minerals. It is important to replace them on the off days

REFERENCES

"A Body in Recovery." Well-Being Oasis. Well-Being-Oasis.com, n.d. Web. 24 April. 2012.

"Herxheimer Reaction." Chronic Illness Recovery Counsel Liason Education. Chronic Illness Recovery, Inc., n.d. Web. 24 April. 2012.

Rull, Gurvinder. "Jarisch-Herxheimer Reaction." Patient.co.uk. EMIS, 1 February 2011. Web. 24 Feb. 2012.

CHAPTER 22

Stress: Don't Let It Wear on You

Stress is actually prolonged worry. It could be worry about job, finances, relationships, or the future. It can exist at a conscious level or an unconscious level. Many people recognize that stress gives them headaches or stomach aches, or even produces ulcers. It can cause the jaw to clench, especially at night during sleep.

But what people don't realize is that stress is a major contributor to all kinds of additional problems in their internal body systems. Stress shuts down various body functions and organs. It constricts the veins and arteries causing high blood pressure and is, in fact, the number one cause of high blood pressure. Research has shown that stress also shrinks the size of the hippocampus, the part of the brain that is responsible for memory and learning.

Prolonged worry or stress turns on the body's flight or fight mechanism—under the control of the sympathetic nervous system—and leaves it on.

Let us take the example of a person encountering a tiger to show how the sympathetic nervous system reacts to stress. At the moment the tiger appears, the person has to quickly make a choice either to stand and fight or to run for dear life. Either way, the fight or flight mechanism kicks in. The heart pumps faster, the arteries to the internal organs constrict and the veins and arteries to the legs and arms dilate to carry more blood and oxygen to the extremities to increase their strength. The digestive tract shuts down so that no energy is diverted to a bodily function that doesn't enhance the chances of surviving the threat. Similarly, the kidneys decrease their output so that the person on the run won't need to pause to void. The adrenal glands pump out more adrenalin and cortisol, and the eyes dilate to bring in more light. When the person is safe and the tiger is no longer a threat, the body returns to its normal function of digesting food, sends blood to the colon and kidney, decreases the heart rate and so forth.

But under prolonged stress the flight or fight mechanism is never switched off. It continues on emergency status, with the result that blood pressure stays high, heart rate stays high, the internal organs suffer for lack of blood and kidney and colon functions remain inhibited. Over time, prolonged stress will cause a breakdown in one of the organs of the body, and the weakest one—or the most toxic one—will fail first.

Many times a person experiencing a constant state of worry becomes so accustomed to it he or she isn't even aware of it anymore. It is possible, especially in the case of a person who experienced severe physical or pschologic trauma as a child, that his or her flight or fight mechanism never shuts down.. He or she is in a constant state of fear of being hurt again. Even later in life, long after the abuse or trauma has stopped, the fear continues and the fight or flight condition stays active because the brain never caught up with the fact that the "tiger" is gone and it's safe now.

It is of major importance to decrease stress in our lives, whether it stems from anger, fear and worry, or the just-too-many-things-to-do syndrome we often find ourselves in, so that we can take things in stride and not wear ourselves out. A study published in the journal Thorax found that hostility and anger reduced lung function over time, independent of other factors such as smoking, and were risk factors for cardiovascular and other diseases. "Stress-related factors are known to depress the immune function and increase susceptibility to or exacerbate a host of diseases and disorders," said Dr Paul Lehrer, of the University of Medicine and Dentistry of New Jersey, in an editorial in the journal.

Ways to decrease stress

There are many ways to decrease stress. Calcium, magnesium and the B vitamins feed the nerves. Increasing magnesium intake will relax tense muscles. Feeding the body B vitamins and trace minerals will support the adrenal glands in their overactivity of producing adrenalin (See Chapter 15).

Young Living's Peace and Calming oil blend calms the brain down and relaxes the body. I enjoy putting a few drops of Peace and Calming, Lavender or Valor oil blend in a nice warm bathtub and taking a bath to relax my muscles or to calm my nervous system. Bathing with these oils relieves a tension headache and stops the stomach from churning. Putting Valor on the forehead and holding one hand over the forehead and the other hand in the back of the head is another good technique for relief of tension headache.

Another way to decrease stress is through simple rest and relaxation. Taking a wonderful, warm bubble bath does wonders to relax the body. Laying out in the sun to read a good book is a nice way to unwind. Going away on vacation is a great way to get away from it all and relax. But it still seems that some people are so wound up about work that even while on vacation relaxation is impossible!

Some great advice from multimillionaire Alex Mandossian is to set a goal of how much money you want to make in 13 weeks. When you reach that goal, drop everything and go on a mini-vacation with the family! He asks what point there is to earning money if not to play?

Meditation and relaxation tapes do wonders to slow the body down. They soothe nerves, calm down brain activity, slow the heart rate and relieve high blood pressure. Meditation is a great time to practice biofeedback. Studies have shown that biofeedback is one of the most effective ways to lower blood pressure. One way to do this is to get to a relaxed state of mind and then imagine all your muscles going limp, one at a time. Start from your head and neck and go all the way to your toes. Then imagine your heart beating at a relaxed and normal rate. Imagine dilated veins and arteries and normal blood flow.

Biofeedback is a powerful method for dealing with stress. I was taught how to do biofeedback at an event where we were to walk on coals. We began by spending a couple of hours imagining our feet being encased in ice. We could feel the ice and feel the chill of our feet. We also imagined that our feet could still sweat profusely in this cold state and that they were in fact dripping wet. It worked! My feet felt so cold they were numb, yet I was in tropical Cancun, Mexico at the time. I was able to walk across the coals without feeling any heat until the last step when I lost my concentration and felt the last coal. The only burn I got was when I lost my focus. If you can learn to do biofeedback you will be able to tone down excess tension at will.

A fundamental and far-too-often-ignored way to control stress is by exercising. Getting a daily workout is fabulous for lowering tension and rebuilding mental and physical perspective. The muscles love exercise.

These techniques work really well for stress caused by conscious problems but, as I said earlier, there may be stress arising from the subconscious, as in the case of a person who has been sexually abused and repressed the memory and associated emotions for their own psyche's protection. In this case, it is important to allow the feelings to finally express themselves and come out in the open where they can be acknowledged and released. There are many emotional release techniques that can help with this, including cranial-sacral, BEST, Return to Freedom and others.

In chapter 13 we talked about cleansing the brain and the limbic system. The limbic system is the emotional center of the brain. Sometimes a memory loop doesn't get turned off in the brain and it just keeps playing the same memory, self-talk or emotion over and over, prolonging stress. The body never gets the message that it is safe from the tiger. People who suppress their emotions and never allow themselves to feel them have this kind of memory loop problem. Emotions are energy in motion and are meant to be felt. Until they are felt to their fullest and then consciously changed, they continue to create trouble, either by distorting body systems or by replaying over and over in the mind.

Releasing emotions

Some people do not believe that you need to feel the emotion to let it go. I have seen many techniques that mask over the emotion but in my experience an emotion that is merely suppressed is not gone but seems to keep manifesting in some way. The emotional techniques that create the most healing are those that let the person feel their emotions, and consciously make a decision to let them go and change how they feel.

Using emotional release techniques with my clients, I have found that forgiveness is the key to healing. Forgiveness does not imply that what the other person did to hurt you was right or okay. Forgiveness simply releases the emotional trauma that you are holding. It assists you to move on with your life without the constant energy demands of having to continually and repeatedly hate someone or feel victimized by what happened. You let go of that and leave it with God so you can live your life unencumbered with what is past and gone. And by choosing to forgive and forget you no longer have an emotional link to the person who hurt you.

I once heard in a psychology lecture that it is important to feel an emotion to its utmost, and then decide if that is how you still want to feel. If it isn't, decide how you do want to feel. Emotions are a choice! They can change depending on our decisions. If you don't want to feel sad anymore, choose some other emotion such as joy, or peace or forgiveness. Doing this stops the memory loop in the brain, relaxes the body and decreases stress.

One of the most amazing programs I have ever witnessed for healing emotional issues is Impact Training. I saw people let go of issues in four days of training that otherwise took months and weeks and sometimes years of emotional release work to get rid of. And those issues remained 'gone.' The people coming out of this training were able to live better, happier, more functional lives. You can find out more about Impact Training at their website at www.impacttrainings.com.

Several essential oil blends do an amazing job of helping to release long-held emotions that are difficult to deal with. The oils go straight to the limbic system of the brain creating a chemical change that releases long-held traumas. They also assist in changing an emotion to one that the person would rather feel.

Here is how I use essential oils to release emotions: I first use Release and 3 Wise Men to bring up the half-buried emotion that I am feeling so that I can really feel it strongly. Usually this brings up the cause or memory of why I am having that emotion. If I deserve a good cry, I cry. If I deserve a good temper tantrum then I throw one. In other words, I allow the negative energy to leave my body. When I am done and ready to change, I use Forgiveness oil and forgive myself for having sent a negative vibration into the world, and to help me forgive the person who offended me, which caused me to create that negative emotion. Then I ask God to forgive me and to forgive the other person as well.

(I read once in a Chinese medicine book that the way to truly heal was to first believe in some type of God ; then forgive your mother for anything that she did to cause your illness; and finally, forgive her doctor since he was advising her on how best to care for you in the only way he knew how. I think that is excellent advice.)

After I have done that, I choose the emotion I would rather feel about the incident in question and I smell the essential oil that names that emotion until it becomes reality. What happens then is that if the painful memory ever comes up again it is no longer associated with the emotion it used to carry with it. The memory might come up again in connection with another emotion, hence the admonition to forgive 70 times 7. For example, I had a certain memory come up several times but with different emotions attached each time. There was horror, terror, hatred, anger, embarrassment and sadness. I had to clear each of those emotions one at a time. When you have cleared all the emotions associated with a memory it will often simply disappear forever, and if it doesn't it won't traumatize you anymore when it does come up. You might even be able to look at it as a great learning opportunity instead of a trauma.

One thing to consider when using essential oils is that emotions are energy vibrations. Like any energy form they send out frequency waves. In physics, to cancel out an energy wave, you send the opposite wave at it with the same amplitude and frequency. A sine wave is negated by a cosine wave of the same amplitude and frequency.

Similarly, to negate an emotion, you send an opposite emotion at it. Sometimes I use a thesaurus to find an antonym of the negative emotion I am feeling. For example, in the past I have sometimes felt fear. So I wrote down a sentence expressing the source of that fear, such as:

"I feel fear when…"
"Selling my house makes me feel afraid that…"
"I am afraid that no one will like me when…."

Then I rewrite the sentence using the antonym:

"I choose to trust that…"
"I choose to feel courage about…,"
"I choose to feel love because, …"
"I choose to feel faith in order to…" etc.

Then I breathe in the oil associated with that positive feeling. For example, Valor blend gives the feeling of courage or faith or trust. Joy blend gives the feeling of love. Peace and Calming blend gives a feeling of calm or peace. Just looking at the name of the blends pretty much tells you how to use it.

When a person is doing an organ cleanse he or she may begin to have memories come back of past hurts or angers. It is important to decide then and there to deal with these old emotions in healthier ways so that they will dissipate. However, sometimes the organ you are cleansing doesn't seem to heal no matter what you do. This is the time to see whether the cause of the organ dysfunction is emotional in nature rather than physical.

In her book, Heal Your Life, Louise Hay has several pages that tell what emotions go with different disease states and with different organs. You can look up the organ that is giving you trouble and see whether the emotion associated with it is similar to what you have experienced. If so, use the appropriate essential oils to release that emotion.

She also has positive affirmations that go along with each organ. It is helpful to smell the oil that goes along with the affirmations while repeating them ten times each. A friend of mine took 15 years off her face by repeating an affirmation from <u>Heal Your Life</u> ten times a day for a week. Every week she did a new affirmation until she had done all of them in the book.

Cleansing the body from the inside out is the way to a more radiant life. Cleansing the physical body and then the emotions, creates "inner transformations" that begin to glow outwardly. It lights the face and can be seen by everyone. Not only do you look more radiant but you feel more radiant. Life has been added to your life. You will be amazed at how many burdens are lifted from your shoulders when you learn to de-stress and to let go of negative emotions.

Case History #1

My story of reversing Fibromyalgia and Chronic Fatigue Syndrome involved healing my spiritual body as well as my physical body. Being a survivor of abuse, I harbored a lot of anger and blame. For years I had the desire to forgive after I heard a professional life strategist describe how forgiveness is a gift you give yourself. It is a gift to decide "I will no longer let this control me." I had no control over the events when they occurred, but I did have control over whether I woke up each day deciding whether I would let them debilitate me or not.

The day I learned my daughter was molested was the day I finally moved from the desire to forgive to the actual decision to forgive. I didn't want her life debilitated by anger and blame like mine had been. I knew Young Living's Seventh Heaven kit would assist me in connecting to this ability so I had it overnighted to our home.

I placed White Angelica across our shoulders, Sacred Mountain on the crowns of our heads, Inspiration over the kidneys (bottom ribs on the back), Humility on the center of the forehead, Dream Catcher on the hairline of the neck, Awaken dragged from the right temple to the left temple, and Gathering on our wrists and temples. We also took the time to smell each of the opened bottles.

For me, these oils lifted the negative energy that distorts rational thinking. I felt like my brain and heart were given a clean slate to write on. Because the heaviness of the negative energy was gone, I was easily able to make a strategy to live by. I decided that abuse didn't give me an exemption from participating in my life. I could no longer place the blame of my crappy life on my abusers. I was fully responsible for how I let those events control me. Every time the past would sneak into my thoughts, I quickly replaced them with healthy ones. In the first two months I had to do this often because I was reprogramming the "tapes" which played over and over in my mind. I got good at catching my thoughts and redirecting them. Because I reprogrammed my thoughts, the past no longer creeps into my awareness.

This was the last key piece needed to remove the "electricity" that jolted through my spine, and to soften my hardened muscles. I had changed my diet and used Super Cal, Sulfurzyme, JuvaCleanse and Raindrop Technique to remove the physical toxins which contributed to FM and CFS. But the Seventh Heaven kit was vital to assist me in removing the emotional toxins I had harbored in my cells. My hardened attitude had hardened my body. I realized that I was chronically fatigued as a result of chronically eating junk and chronically taxing my body with emotional stress. The body has an amazing ability to regenerate and heal itself when given the proper tools to do so. I now live a beautiful, joyful life thanks to the pure healing power of these oils. Because of this new example, my daughter does too.

Tiffany Rowan
Little Rock, Arkansas

Case History #2

I love it when God gives me signs I can actually understand! As I was meditating this morning on my recent colon-cleansing experience I was visually shown my life as a 'slate' (as in 'washing the slate clean') and I saw that only 1/4 of the slate was white, pristine, clean and ready to receive entirely new information. (Interesting after this 1st deep cleanse, I cleaned out everything in about a 1/4 of my colon right down to the colon wall where new and healthy cells are growing fresh and pristine for the first time since I was born). Then I saw that the other 3/4 of the slate was covered in layers upon layers of creations...each layer built on top of the other and piled high. It was a mass of creation...not bad, not good...just was the accumulation of everything I have done in my life up to now. (Very much like the condition of the rest of my colon). And, I could see very clearly what I was being inspired to understand over the past 3 years....that I now have a space in my life on which to truly create something fresh and new or I can choose to leave it blank and eventually what I have been doing will simply take over that space and I will continue to get more of the same as what I have had. And, what I have has been great. Yet, I have been praying to God for more wellness, more energy, more prosperity, more loving spirit because the old way of doing has only gotten me so far. So, the space has been created. I will continue to pray and meditate and breathe until I receive the next inspiration about what to grow in this rich and fertile soil.

Stacy Hall,
Author, *Chi-To-Be*

To me this is what cleansing is all about, becoming physically and spiritually purified and adding "Life to Your Life" to be able to be a more radiant you; having a clean temple in which God can dwell.

—LD—

REFERENCES

Lupien SJ, Fiocco A, Wan N, Maheu F, Lord C, Schramek T, Tu MT. Stress hormones and human memory function across the lifespan. Psychoneuroendocrinology. 2005 Apr;30(3):225-42

Guyton, Arthur C., Textbook of Medical Physiology, WB Saunders Company, Philadelphia PA 1991

Laura D Kubzansky, David Sparrow, Benita Jackson, Sheldon Cohen, Scott T Weiss, and Rosalind J Wright. Angry breathing: a prospective study of hostility and lung function in the Normative Aging Study. Thorax, Sep 2006; doi:10.1136/thx.2005.050971

Garrison Jr., Robert H. & Elizabeth Somer, The Nutrition Desk Reference. Keats Publishing, Inc. New Canaan CT 1990

Hay, Louise, Heal Your Life, Hay House, Inc. Carlsbad, CA. 1984

AFTERWORD AND QUICK REFERENCE GUIDE

Now that you have cleansed your body, whether for the first time or not, it would be a good idea to cleanse regularly. I suggest you use the seasons of the year as a guide to your cleansing program. Using the seasons to cleanse each organ will keep your body in top-notch working order. Below is a quick reference guide to remind you when to clean each system.

Fall: Colon, lungs, skin
Winter: Kidney, bones, yeast
Early Spring: Master Cleanse, liver, ligaments
Late Spring: early summer: gall bladder
Early Summer: small intestines, heart, circulation, endocrine system
Late Summer: stomach, spleen, muscles

Here is a step by step process of the methods described in this book. Though I recommend doing each cleanse in the correct season, if you have never cleansed, just start now and cleanse in this order:

FALL

1. Colon cleanse: Start with 1 Comfortone and build up to 10 daily. Take 2 Essentialzyme between meals. Take 2 Detoxzyme as needed for toxicity. Start ICP as soon as you are having at least 2 bowel movements a day. Stay on the colon cleanse for the remainder of the cleanses.

2. After a week or two of being on the colon cleanse, cleanse the kidney by using K&B (from Dr. Christopher), Juniper, Sage, and Rosemary. You can

do this for a week or two before you start the Master Cleanse, since the Master Cleanse also cleans the kidney.

3. If you have a yeast problem it is often better to do a yeast cleanse before the Master Cleanse. Use Melrose, Stevia extract, and acidophilus to clear yeast.

WINTER

4. You need to be having 3 good bowel movements daily to start with Master Cleanse diet. Follow instructions exactly. Do the Master Cleanse for at least 10 days. Stay on Comfortone, use 3 drops Peppermint oil in the morning and 3 at night. Do the salt water drink in the morning. Drink it as quick as you can. (I recommend only doing the salt water 2 or 3 times a week. If you get runny stools, use ½ tsp ICP at night to help thicken the stools.) (See the book "Healing for the Age of Enlightenment") and go back to Essentialzyme (if you have not dropped the mucoid plaque) and Detoxyme as needed.

5. One week after completing the Master Cleanse, go on Parafree to get rid of parasites.

SPRING

6. Begin a liver cleanse at this point using Juva Cleanse, JuvaTone and the Re-JUVA-Nate protocol of juice fasting. I highly recommend staying on this cleanse for at least 4 months, preferably 6 months.

7. Continue colon cleansing until the lining of the bowel (mucoid plaque) drops out as directed. This may take anywhere from a few weeks to 18 months or more.

8. When the lining of the bowel comes out, begin reducing the Comfortone and ICP until you are off of them to see how your bowel is functioning on its own. If all of your problems have cleared up you can go off the cleanses and see how your body functions. If you feel you still have some things to clear up, continue on with the cleanses.

9. To remain at optimal health the rest of your life after your first major cleanse, take a few weeks with every season of the year to cleanse and build your organ systems as described in this book. If done seasonally you will find that you never again will have to spend months cleansing your body, but just a few weeks out of each season.

While cleansing the body it helps to speed the cleanse along and to assist the organs and tissues to rebuild by using the Organ Balances in my book, "Ultimate Balance" available through Life Science Publishers.

It is an excellent idea to change your diet. As mentioned throughout the book, white flour products and products devoid of nutrition are toxic to the body. Eat as fresh and raw as you possibly can to be able to receive enzymes and vitamins and minerals. Eating fresh fruits and vegetables will also give your body fiber which is necessary to form healthy stools. Eating as many fermented foods such as vegetables and fermented breads and dairy products will add necessary probiotics into the gut. Eat sprouts; they are rich in the B vitamins and enzymes. Cut down on meat. Cut out breads and empty calorie items like cake and cookies etc. Drink more water. Cut out sodas and caffeine drinks. These steps will make huge differences in your health.

Now that you have created an Inner Transformation, don't be surprised if people have asked you what you have done to create such outer radiance!

Cleansing the body restores life to your life! I wish you a long and healthy one!

Quick Reference Guide to various cleanses throughout the book

COLON CLEANSE

1. Begin with 1 ComforTone in the morning. The second day take one in the morning and one in the evening. The third day take two in the morning and one in the evening, then two in the morning and two in the evening and so on, building up to a maximum of 10 daily. Remember that your goal is 2 to 3 bowel movements a day that are fast and easy to pass, well formed and float in the toilet. When you reach that goal you don't need to add any more capsules daily. Stay on that level until you pass the mucoid plaque. If you are having diarrhea, decrease your capsules until your bowels are firm again. If you are having constipation, decrease your capsules until your bowels are easier to pass or add magnesium, peppermint oils or get an adjustment from a chiropractor.

   Along with the ComforTone, take Essentialzyme caplet 3 times daily, between meals. Drink your water!

2. When having 2-3 good bowel movements daily begin taking ICP, 1 tsp in the morning. Mix it with juice and drink it down quickly. Add ½ tsp per day until you reach 1 Tbsp. (3 tsp.) in the morning and 1 Tbsp. in the evening. Stay on ComforTone and Essentialzyme. Keep drinking lots of water!

3. Continue colon cleansing until the mucoid plaque drops out of the colon. This may take between 6 weeks and 18 months. <u>To help speed the cleansing along it is a good idea to use the Large Intestine energy balance from "Ultimate Balance".</u>

 Scan the QR Code to find out more about the mucoid plaque.

LIVER CLEANSE

I suggest you follow one or the other of the following two protocols. The first one is simple but will take more time to completely cleanse the liver.

- Take one JuvaTone pill the first day, adding one pill a day until you get to 5, then keep taking 5 a day for the duration of the cleanse.
- Use 3- 15 drops of Juva Cleanse a day or as needed. (I usually do 3 drops 5 times a day.) "As needed" means for nausea, headaches, stomachaches, gas, aches and pains, etc.
- Stay on this protocol for 4 months, then begin noticing whether your symptoms have gone away. It will probably take longer than 4 months, perhaps up to 18 months.

The second protocol is my favorite. It does take more effort, because you have to make two juices to drink, but it works faster. Drinking these cleansing juices while also taking the Young Living products is easier on the body and makes for a quicker, effective cleanse. I felt better on it, had more energy and had a quicker cleanse. With the juices, the JuvaTone, Juva Cleanse and other supplements, it only takes 4-6 months to clean a liver, whereas the first protocol, above, may take 18 months. You can do modified juicing if you prefer, just drinking the juice a few times a day instead of every hour. That is still effective.

This cleansing protocol is called the Re-JUVA-nate diet. It has been updated a little from the original to incorporate the new products that have been introduced since the time of the first one, and also includes Vital Life juice. Here's how it goes:

- Immediately after you wake up: Drink a 10 oz glass of the special lemonade drink (the recipe is given the daily schedule):
- And take these supplements:
2 JuvaTone
2 Detoxzyme
2 Essentialzyme-4
20 Drops of Juva Cleanse in a capsule (or in a tsp of some nutritious oil, or if you choose to take it directly by mouth, i.e., by applying it to your inner cheek, you only need 3-4 drops 3 times a day.)

- One hour later, drink the Vita Life juice (the recipe is given below, following the lemonade recipe):
- Alternate the lemonade drink with Vita Life juice every hour throughout the day.
- For lunch eat a salad with 1 tablespoon Juva Power mixed in.
- Drink a glass of Powermeal sometime during the day to sustain you.
- For dinner eat a light meal. Salads, nuts, sprouts, sweet potatoes, nuts, or nut butter, fish or a small amount of poultry, fresh natural grains like quinoa, millet or brown rice and some flaxseed or cod-liver oil are wonderful to keep the liver cleansing. Avoid pork and pork products and fatty red meats.
- And take the same supplements as in the morning:
  2 JuvaTone
  2 Detoxzyme
  2 Essentialzyme-4
  20 Drops of Juva Cleanse in a capsule (or in a tsp of some nutritious oil.)

This is an amazing and powerful Liver Cleanse. Make sure you are still having 2 or 3 bowel movements a day, like you started having with the colon cleanse, to get the toxins released by this cleanse safely out of the body. If you aren't still having 2-3 bowel movements a day, take ICP and Comfortone as directed in Chapter 4 to get back to that condition.

Lemonade drink recipe:
  2 Tbl fresh squeezed lemon juice
  2 Tbl grade B maple syrup
  10 oz purified water
  1/8 tsp cayenne pepper

Vital Life juice recipe:
  3oz beet
  1oz celery
  1oz carrot
  1/3 oz Black Spanish radish (or Daigon Radish or White Radish)
  1/8th oz ginger root
  1/3 oz red potato

KIDNEY CLEANSE

Cleanse the kidney by using K&B (from Dr. Christopher) as directed on the bottle. I like to add K& B a glass of cranberry juice, a ¼ cup of flax seed oil and a drop each of Juniper, RC, Sage, and Rosemary essential oils to the mix. You can do this for a week or two before you start the Master Cleanse. The Master Cleanse does a great job of cleansing the kidney.

SIBO, IBS, IBD, Crohn's and other inflammatory bowel conditions.

1. Go on a paleo diet; above all it must be gluten and free casein free, until you get the gut cleaned up. I recommend that you stay off wheat for about 18 months while clearing up the small and large intestines. Then you can slowly add it back in to see if you still react to it. The inability to digest wheat stems from this inflammation. Wheat interacts with heavy metals and the inflammation causing more inflammation. Casein or milk protein, particularly from pasteurized and homogenized dairy products, creates a lot of mucus in the body, especially since the milk-digesting enzyme has been destroyed in processing.

2. Use the 5-Day Nutritive Cleanse from Young Living. It is not a targeted cleanse, just a support while reducing inflammation. The 5-Day Nutritive Cleanse facilitates gentle and effective cleansing to improve overall health and well-being. YLO says "A minimum of four, easy cleanses a year with our 5-Day Nutritive Cleanse and continued nutritional maintenance will help balance the extremes of the modern diet." This nutritive cleanse includes the following: NingXia Red, an energizing, replenishing, whole wolfberry nutrient infusion (1500 ml); Balance Complete, a super-food-based, daily, superfood energizer and nutritive cleanse (26.4 oz.); and Digest + Cleanse, which soothes gastrointestinal discomfort and supports healthy digestion. Note: The 5-Day Nutritive Cleanse is a starting place. More intense and targeted nutrients may be required for your particular situation. The 5-Day Nutritive Cleanse facilitates gentle and effective cleansing to improve overall health and well-being.

3. It is imperative that you bring down the inflammation of the large and small intestine. While cleansing with the 5-Day Nutritive Cleanse, give yourself rectal injections of Idaho Balsam Fir, Frankincense and Copaiba essential

oils. Also, mix 1-3 drops of those same oils with coconut milk or coconut oil or some other type of fatty oil such as almond oil, cod-liver oil, flax seed oil, olive oil, etc.and either include these oils in smoothies or just ingest them straight. Mixing with a fatty oil will emulsify the essential oil and assist it to bypass the acid of the stomach, allowing it to go straight to the small intestine and be absorbed into the cells there. Those four essential oils are great anti-inflammatory oils. Adding Melaleuca alternifolia will assist in working on the yeast that may be in the small intestine and large intestine. (See the yeast chapter.)

4. I suggest you do the Master Cleanse for at least 10 days, preferably as long as 40 days. While you are on it, you can take ICP and ComforTone to assist you in passing the toxins out of the body. (Read Tom Woloshy's book "Beyond the Master Cleanse" and the Master Cleanse chapter in this book) Continue to use the rectal injections as mentioned above and keep ingesting those same oils in a fatty type oil. I prefer to use coconut oil as it is also a yeast killer itself.

5. When done with the Master Cleanse you will probably be able to start a more targeted colon cleanse in order to assist the colon in being able to function better. Start using the Cleansing Trio Kit by Young Living Oils.

6. It is also extremely important to restore the beneficial bacteria in the body. This can be done in by eating fermented foods and taking Life 5 or another good probiotic. There are many websites that teach how to ferment your foods online, or you can just buy apple cider vinegar, yogurt, kefir and so forth. Life 5 is an amazing probiotic. Balance Complete also has pectin in it, which has been shown to feed the beneficial bacteria in the colon.

7. You may also want to remove metals from the body while you are cleansing with the Cleansing Trio Kit.

METAL CLEANSE
A powerful, no-holds-barred metal cleanse

Here is a complete metal cleansing protocol. This cleanse picks up heavy metals, cleanses the liver, clears lymph, cleanses the kidney, and supports the spleen and adrenal glands. You want to have done colon and kidney cleanses before this starting this metal cleanse, and preferably a Master Cleanse as well, to make sure the metals and toxins have a clear path to the exit.

This cleanse is a potent detoxifier. However, if you feel like you are detoxing too heavily, I urge you to use more JuvaCleanse and Detoxyme frequently throughout the day. Note that this cleanse is a 3-day repeating cycle.

DAY 1—Mobilizes metals.

* **First thing in morning upon arising:**
    Drink water
    Follow that with a tall glass of the following detoxifying lemonade drink:

    LEMONADE DRINK
    2 Tbl fresh squeezed lemon juice
    2 Tbl grade B maple syrup
    10 oz purified water
    1/8 tsp cayenne pepper

    And take these supplements:
    2 JuvaTone
    1 Comfortone
    2 Detoxzyme
    2 Essentialzyme-4
    2 L-Methionine 500 Mg
    1 Super B
    20 Drops of Juva Cleanse in a capsule (or if you choose to take it directly by mouth, i.e., by applying it to your inner cheek, you only need 3-4 drops, but do it 5 or 6 times a day.)

- **9 am**

  Do the spleen balance found in Ultimate Balance book. Use one of the oils listed in Ultimate Balance for spleen (i.e., Surrender, Release, Gratitude, Hope or Thieves)

  Drink 8 oz. fresh pineapple/grapefruit juice to clear spleen and lymph glands. **Add 2 drops of Grapefruit™ essential oil to the juice.**

- **10:45**

  Repeat spleen balance in Ultimate Balance

- **Lunch**

  Drink Powermeal or Pure Protein Complete, ideally in some sort of fatty liquid, coconut milk, kefir, yogurt, etc. Add 4 drops of Frankincense, 4 drops of Copaiba, and 4 drops of Helichrysum, essential oils to the fatty liquid. The cream or fat in the liquid will mix with the oils and help them past the stomach acid into the small intestine.

  Eat a salad with 1 tablespoon Juva Power mixed in.

  Take 2 Essentialzyme-4

  Drink 1 tablespoon ICP in juice and 2 oz NingXia Red (Drink NingXia Red throughout the day for blood sugar issues as needed.)

  Also have some cilantro pesto. Eat it plain or mix in the salad or eat as a vegetable dip.

  CILANTRO PESTO
  1 bunch cilantro, washed & dried
  3 cloves garlic
  1/2 c. olive oil
  1/2 tsp. salt
  1/2 tsp. pepper
  1/4 c. pine nuts (or another soft nut such as walnut or cashew)
  2 drops of Helichrysum essential oil
  3 drops of Coriander essential oil
  Mix ingredients in food processor until smooth.

- **1 pm**

  Do the small intestine energy balance in the UItimate Balance book using one or more essential oils as listed in the book. (Hope, DiGize, Purification, Harmony, Peppermint)

- **2 pm**

  Drink Vital Life juice:

  VITAL LIFE JUICE

  3oz beet

  1oz celery

  1oz carrot

  1/3 oz Black Spanish radish (or Daigon radish or white radish)

  1/8th oz ginger root

  1/3 oz red potato

  4 oz cilantro

  1 bud of garlic

  2 drops of Coriander™ essential oil

  All of the above in a blender. Please weigh the vegetables! If you use too much you can get very toxic.

  Alternate the lemonade you made in the morning with this Vital Life juice every hour throughout the day as needed for detox or hunger. Eat Pesto also as needed for hunger.

- **2:45 pm**

  Repeat small intestine balance.

  Have some kefir or yogurt with a drop or two of Melrose, Frankincense, Copaiba or Helichrysum mixed in it.

- **5 pm**

  Do the kidney balance from Ultimate Balance with Juniper and Valor. Use K&B as needed.

  Eat a small dinner. Fish is best. Have more cilantro pesto and a salad with Power Meal. No wheat or gluten products

- **6:45 pm**

  Repeat kidney balance.

  Continue to alternate Vital Life juice and the lemonade juice as needed for hunger or detoxing.

- **9 pm and again at 10:45pm if you are awake**

  Do the adrenal balance in Ultimate Balance, using one of the oils listed (Nutmeg, Endoflex, Hope, Surrender or Clove)

DAY 2—Detox day.

Eat fermented vegetables to bind metals and carry them out via the colon, use 1 Detoxyzme between meals, jump start Juva Cleanse as needed throughout the day. These will pull the metals you have mobilized out of the body. Eat normal meals, but no wheat or gluten products. Take Mineral Essence as directed on the bottle.

DAY 3—Rest day

Just eat normally again but no wheat or gluten products. (If needed, take the same detox supplements and oils as Day 2.) Take Mineral Essence as directed on the bottle.

DAY 4—A repeat of Day 1.

Begin to mobilize metals again and continue this cycle.

This is an amazing and very powerful liver cleanse and metal cleanse!

APPENDIX A

Vita Flex Foot Chart

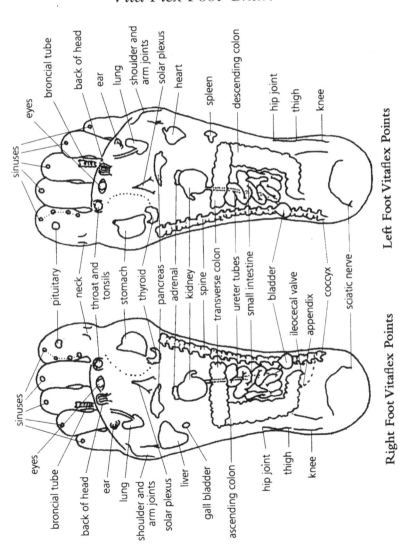

Organ Alarm Points

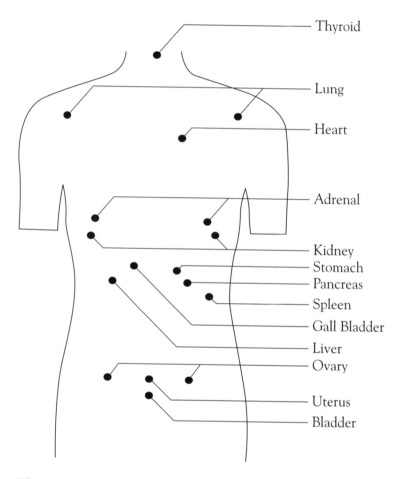

The adrenal and kidney points are on the back.

Small intestine and Large intestine points are tested by placing the palm down over the navel area then over the lower abdomen.

The Pituitary Point is between the eyes at the bridge of the nose

APPENDIX B

Organs and Essential Oils

Adrenals:
Mineral Essence
Nutmeg
Prenolone +
Super B
OmegaGize
Cortistop

Colon:
Comfortone
ICP
Essentialzyme
Detoxzyme
Di-Gize
Peppermint
Life-5

Gallbladder
GLF
Juva Tone
Life-5

Hormones, Mens:
Mister
Goldenrod
Protec
Prenolone +
Super B
OmgaGize
Clove
Nutmeg
Prostate Health

Hormones, Womens:
Progessence +
Prenolone +
Femigen
Clary Sage
Dragon Time
Sclaressence
Bergamot
Estro

Kidney:
K&B
Juniper
Valor
Sage
Geranium

Liver:
Juva Cleanse
Juva Tone
Juva Flex
GLF
(Release- emotional)
(Forgiveness -
emotional)
Essentialzymes-4

Lungs:
Raven or
Ravintsara
Thyme
RC
Oregano
Peppermint

Muscles
Release
Marjoram
Aroma Siez
Relieve It
Super B
Super Cal
Regenolone
Mineral Essence
Sulferzyme

Nervous System:
Mega Cal
Super B
Mineral Essence
Peace and Calming
Feelings Kit
Tranquil Roll-on
Stress Away
Valor
Progessence +
(Women)
Cortistop

Pancreas:
Stevia
Thieves
Sulferzyme
New NingXia Red
Coriander
Essentialzymes-4
Dill
Ocotea

PH
Alkalime

Pituitary:
Ultra Young + Spray
Sacred Frankincense
Blue Cypress
Idaho Balsam Fir
Lavender

Spleen:
ImmuPower
3 Wisemen
ImmuPro
Rehemogen
Grapefruit
Ledum

Stomach:
Di-Gize
Peppermint
Alkalime
Ginger
Fennel

Thyroid:
Endoflex
Myrtle
Lemongrass
Thyromin

APPENDIX C

Enzymes

Let's talk a little about enzymes. First, what are enzymes? These amazing complex molecules are catalysts; in other words, they make chemical reactions happen, or happen much faster than they otherwise would. As such, they are an extremely important part of your body physiology. Active in every cell of the body, thousands of unique enzymes together constitute the stuff that makes things happen, different enzymes being found in different cells, depending on the function of that cell. Life as we know it could not exist without the constant activity of our enzymes.

For our purposes here, we are interested in digestive enzymes, those that help us digest the various things we take into our bodies. Our bodies create enzymes that help us digest proteins, others that work on carbohydrates, and others that are specific for fats. They are created in the stomach, the small intestine, the liver and the pancreas – even in the mouth. Proper digestion would simply not be possible without the enzymes found in our digestive tract and thus we would derive no nutrition from our food.

Unfortunately, due to various factors such as age or illness, for example, our bodies sometimes fail to produce enough enzymes to do the job of digesting everything we eat. Foods acquired in nature come with their own enzymes that help with their digestion, but the highly unnatural foods that we commonly pick up at the supermarket usually have been grown with chemical fertilizers and pesticides, subjected to heat in processing, modified beyond all recognition, and pasteurized or sterilized. As a result, they have lost their natural enzymes, making the job of digestion more difficult or even impossible for our bodies. As a result, we end up with sludgy, slow, sick bowels, organs that cannot carry out their proper functions, and poor nutrition. Other signs of digestive enzyme deficiency include fatigue, heartburn, gas, constipation, yeast infections and eczema, to name just a few.

We may also take in substances that the body was not designed to digest, for which it does not naturally make useful enzymes, including genetically-modified (GMO) foods, and food additives. These things, not found in nature, add to the burden on our organs. In addition, the body's enzymes can be rendered ineffective by other molecules called inhibitors. These may enter our body by way of drugs, heavy metals and environmental toxins. Besides interfering with enzymatic activity, they are indigestible and difficult to eliminate from the body. Thus cleansing is critical, and enzymes are essential.

Here is where Young Living enzyme products come in; assisting us to digest the unnatural foods that have been stripped of whatever enzymes they may have had originally. Each product is formulated for a specific purpose, but they overlap in their usefulness.

Allerzyme is a complex, vegetarian blend of enzymes and essential oils designed to combat allergies and problems arising from poor bowel function, such as gas, fermentation, poor absorption, water retention and irritable bowel syndrome. In addition to a powerful array of essential oils, it contains enzymes that help break down proteins, sugars, starches and fats, and to make minerals more available. The name Allerzyme reflects the fact that 80 percent of the immune system is in the gut.

Detoxzyme is a combination of essential oils that work to detoxify and cleanse the digestive system, including the liver and the gallbladder duct, together with specific enzymes to help digest fats, starches and proteins. It also contains phytase to promote absorption of important minerals found in nuts, seeds and grains. In addition, Detoxyme may help keep down cholesterol and triglyceride levels as well as candida/yeast overgrowth.

Essentialzyme is aimed at the reduction of mucus buildup throughout the body and the elimination of toxic waste. The enzymes in Essentialzyme are particularly vital for anyone who has reduced or blocked pancreatic or gallbladder function, acting to restore proper enzyme balance. With its wide array of enzymes, essential oils and botanical ingredients, it helps promote digestion, re-establishment of beneficial flora in the gut and elimination of toxic waste.

Essentialzymes-4 is actually a combination of three former Young Living products: Carbozyme, Lypozyme and Polyzyme. As such, it combines the actions of those products to assist in digesting carbohydrates, fats, and proteins found in modern overly-processed foods and promote the absorption of nutrients for increased vitality. It incorporates dual-time release of enzymes at appropriate phases of the digestive process for enhanced effectiveness.

Any of these products will help digestion and improve nutrition. If you don't have the one that is most indicated for your condition, "in case of fire, break glass." In other words, use what you have.

APPENDIX D

Gall Bladder Flush

I almost hate to include this in the book. That is why I chose to put it in as an appendix, hidden away in the back of the book. Many people have gone on gall bladder flushes over the years. There is a lot of controversy about them. One hears stories of stuck gall stones from a gall bladder flush, but the stories are always second- or third-hand. In chiropractic school we were taught to never advise anyone to do a gall bladder flush, just in case a gallstone does get stuck, which would lead to emergency surgery. So after being apprised of all that, you are fully forewarned that there could be problems with a gall bladder flush. There are many recipes on the internet for these flushes. Below you will find the one that I did 15 years ago and could never bring myself to do again. I include it here only because I mentioned it in the book and people always ask me about it. I found it painful to pass the stones, I had a lot of cramping, I felt every stone leaving and I thought that I had died when I passed out on the floor! Now if I feel the need to flush out the gall bladder I use Grapefruit oil and Ledum and Juvaflex as described in the book. It's much less painful and it seems to be very effective.

7 Day Gall Bladder Flush

Eat 6-7 apples a day or drink 5-6 glasses of freshly made organic apple juice every day for seven days. You can continue to eat normally while doing this but I prefer to do a fast.

On day seven, do an enema in the morning. That night, an hour before retiring, drink 1 tablespoon Epsom salts dissolved in 6 oz. of distilled water. Cool water helps it go down easier. About an hour later, right at bedtime, drink ½ cup of olive oil and ¼ cup of fresh squeezed lemon juice in 8 oz of distilled water. It works best to alternate the two drinks. Be sure to brush your teeth with baking soda to neutralize the acid of drinking the lemon juice.

Go straight to bed, lying on your stomach or in the runner's position. In either position pull your right knee fully upwards, towards your right shoulder, trying to stay as much on your stomach as you can. A pillow under your left shoulder will help. Now relax into this position, and then shift your weight to your right side. Keep your right knee held fully upwards to your chest for 30 minutes. The expulsion of the gall stones happens at this time. After the 30 minutes has passed you can relax, change positions and go to sleep. If any nausea or acid-reflux is felt during the night, get up and immediately take some Peppermint oil or some Juvaflex in water.

In the morning, give yourself another enema to make sure that all the toxins are clear from the colon. Some recipes call for coffee enemas. I think that adding 7 drops of Juvaflex to the enema would work to open the gall bladder and liver ducts.

Drink 2 tablespoons of Epsom salts dissolved in 6 oz. water. About a half hour later drink 8 oz of fresh squeezed orange juice or grapefruit juice.

Some recipes call for doing the flush 4-6 times more over the course of several months.

I myself would rather use the methods described in Chapter 11 under the heading Gall Bladder.

APPENDIX E

Cold Sheet Treatment

This is a wonderful treatment for pneumonia and other lung congestions as well as sinus congestion. It may not be that pleasant to do, but when all else fails, this works. The original recipe given below lists herbs and herbal teas, but you can substitute the appropriate essential oils.

You'll need:
- Peppermint tea (or catnip, thyme and sage, feverfew or red raspberry); enough for at least 4 cups
- Peppermint tea again (or yarrow, boneset, thyme, catnip or similar); at least a cup or two
- Garlic, 10 cloves
- Apple cider vinegar or lemon juice, 1 cup
- More vinegar for washing
- Cayenne pepper, ground mustard, ginger; 3 Tbs each
  Petroleum jelly; at least ½ cup
- Old cloths that you can throw away after wrapping the feet in them
- One sheet
- A bathtub
- A sheet of plastic large enough to cover your mattress

Step one: Give an enema of 4 cups cold peppermint tea (or catnip, thyme and sage, feverfew or red raspberry)

Step two: Give another enema of 3-4 finely grated cloves of garlic mixed into 1 cup apple cider vinegar and 1 cup cold water. (I personally cannot handle the vinegar so I use lemon juice instead.) This is an important step as it strips the mucus from the entire body, but it is also painful. Retain this enema as long as possible. A slant board helps. It is easier to pass the garlic through a syringe than an enema tube, but if you are doing this treatment on yourself it means having someone assist you with this step.

Step three: HOT bath. In an old nylon stocking put 3 Tbs each of cayenne pepper, ground mustard and ginger. (It's best to use all three but use what you have.) Put the stocking in the hot bathwater and get in the tub. Drink peppermint tea while in the bath. If you don't have peppermint tea, you can use these teas instead: yarrow, boneset, thyme, catnip, etc. (Thyme is great for lungs.) Stay in the tub at least half an hour, longer if possible. The purpose of this step is to sweat.

Step four: Wrap a cold wet sheet around the patient. Lay on a bed (use a plastic sheet to protect the mattress). Spread a mixture of petroleum jelly and chopped garlic (about 6 bulbs) on the soles of the feet. It takes about one half cup of petroleum jelly to spread it 1/2 inch thick on the soles of the feet. Wrap cloths around the feet and hold them on with safety pins or slip old socks over the cloths. Cover up with a dry cotton sheet and natural fiber blankets and stay there all night.

Step five: In the morning wipe off the Vaseline and garlic and wash the body with a half and half mixture of vinegar and water.

Remember, I offer this as a suggestion only. The FDA has not approved this treatment and I am not permitted to say or imply that it cures anything.

APPENDIX F

The Limbic System

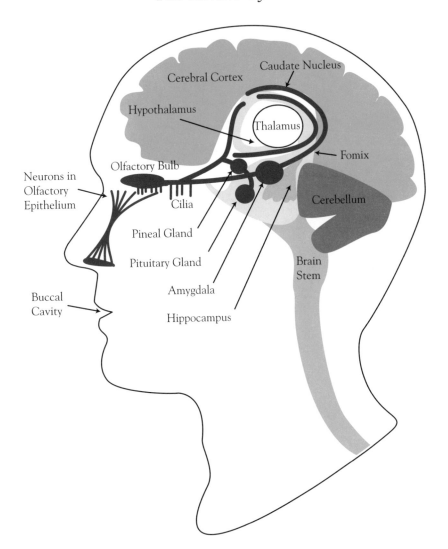

Cerebral Cortex

Caudate Nucleus

Hypothalamus

Thalamus

Fomix

Olfactory Bulb

Neurons in
Olfactory
Epithelium

Cilia

Cerebellum

Pineal Gland

Pituitary Gland

Brain
Stem

Amygdala

Buccal
Cavity

Hippocampus

INDEX

pathogens: 45, 223
Peace and Calming: 22, 53-54, 121, 137-138, 141,
    158, 188, 226, 230, 250
penny: 65
Peppermint: 20-22, 31, 33-34, 68-69, 71, 73-74, 85,
    94, 107, 114-115, 117, 137, 186, 188-190, 196,
    200, 209, 222, 236, 238, 245, 249-250, 256-258
peppermint tea: 71, 114, 257-258
pepsin: 26
peristalsis: 27-28, 33
pernicious anemia: 132
pertussis: 23
pesticides: 2, 21, 76, 81, 169, 223, 251
Pfieffer: 3
pH: 9, 12, 17, 42, 58, 66-67, 87, 120, 134, 138, 142,
    212, 250
phosphoric: 50
phosphorus: 91, 180, 219
pituitary: iv, 143-145, 154, 163, 172, 176-177, 214,
    250
plants: 3, 9, 12, 19-21, 43-44, 76, 80, 90, 144, 160,
    169, 223
plaque: 28, 31, 33-34, 68, 71, 104-105, 125, 236,
    238
pleurisy: 135, 137
pollutant: 89
Polyzyme: 138, 252
potassium: 52, 54, 73, 89, 102, 105, 151, 179-180,
    219
potato: 83, 95, 194, 205, 240, 245
Power Meal: 87, 95, 245
prebiotics: 42, 44
pregnancy: 126, 138, 153, 155, 158, 163-164, 168-
    170, 172-174, 176-177, 181-183, 193, 270
pregnenolone: 155
Prenolone: 155-157, 174, 249
Present Time: 125, 201
probiotics: 2, 44-46, 61-62, 65, 97, 137, 237
Progessence: vii, 155-158, 164, 174, 249-250
Progessence Plus: vii, 174
progesterone: 18, 138, 152, 155-156, 176
prostate: 8, 162-163, 165, 249
proteins: 6, 13, 26, 29, 49-50, 54, 56, 58, 72, 75, 81,
    100, 104, 106-107, 116, 138, 155, 170, 195, 197,
    205, 208, 213, 217-219, 251-253
prunasin: 3
psoriasis: 77, 116, 170, 209
psyllium seed,: 31, 42
purification oil: 65, 85, 92, 125, 204
pyloric valve: 26
questionnaire: 7-8
quinoa: 64, 83, 240
radiant: 0, c, xi, 16, 231, 233
radish: 83, 94, 240, 245
rage: 4, 17
raindrop technique: 54, 121, 122, 131, 137, 232
rash: 64, 118, 146, 190, 197, 209
Rashes: 35, 77, 116, 135, 170-171, 173, 189, 208-
    209, 211, 222
Ravensara: 189

RC: 115-117, 137, 190-191, 209, 241, 249
rebound: 116
receptor sites: 64, 67, 99, 147, 169, 204
Rectal Injection: 181, 195, 200
Reference Guide: iv, 235, 238
reflexology: 21-22, 137
Rehemogen: 123, 132, 210, 250
revenge: 17
rose oil: 20-21
Rosemary: 23, 31, 52, 54, 137, 235, 241
royal medical society: 29
Royaldophilus: 61
sad: 5, 205-206, 217, 228
sage: 23, 52, 54, 137, 156, 158, 183, 235, 241, 249, 257
saline: 116, 209
saliva: 26, 59
salt: vii, 5, 54-56, 65, 68-69, 72, 94, 103, 116, 175,
    188, 219, 222, 236, 244
salt water: 68-69, 236
Sandalwood: 135, 137-138
Schultz, Dr. Susan: 206
Sclaressence: 137-138, 152, 156, 183, 249
scoliosis: x, 131
sea salt: 68
season: iii, 11-16, 99, 121, 191, 211, 235, 237
seizures: 90, 135, 137
senna: 71
sex drive: 8, 77, 157
shampoos: 76, 185
SHED: 12, 206
shoulders: 17, 130-131, 231
SIBO: 108-109, 200, 241
sine wave: 230
sinus: 21, 115, 119, 190-191, 209, 223, 257
sinusitis: 58, 115, 208-209, 211
skin: v-vi, x, 4, 7-8, 15, 20, 22, 24, 30, 35, 45, 56,
    58, 67, 73-74, 76-78, 103, 108, 113, 116-120,
    135-138, 140, 146-148, 156, 163, 169-171, 174-
    175, 178, 185-190, 193, 198, 208-209, 211, 218,
    222, 235
slivers: 119
small intestine: vii, xi, 12, 15, 25-27, 92, 94-95,
    106-109, 155, 175, 200, 241-242, 244-245, 251
smell: v, 22, 52, 54, 96, 115, 119, 141, 156, 183,
    187-188, 229, 231
Smoothies: 215, 242
soaps: 2, 76, 117, 185
soda pop: 50, 206
spine: v, 17, 105, 121-122, 124, 131, 149, 183, 192,
    194, 232
spleen: xi, 12-13, 15, 92-93, 99-100, 112, 199, 214,
    221, 235, 243-244, 250
spring: iii, xi, 12-15, 49, 75, 78, 84-85, 99, 109, 113,
    211, 235-236
starches: 13, 26, 29, 81, 133, 175, 252
stevia: 63-65, 133, 137, 236, 250
stomach: xi, 7, 12, 15, 17, 21, 26-27, 32, 52, 56,
    69, 85, 94, 103, 106-109, 119, 133, 155, 180,
    189-190, 195, 214, 223, 225, 227, 235, 242, 244,
    250-251, 256

"Dr. LeAnne is wise and intuitive. Her stories and sense of humor make complex issues easy to understand."

—Rebecca Bentley-Perez

"Dr. LeAnne is truly an inspiration, she doesn't just talk about it, she walks the walk. She truly has a love for people and desires them to be healthy."

—Maija Laitinen Sevigny

"After spending thousands of dollars, trying to find out where many of my symptoms were coming from, Dr. LeAnne Deardeuff walked me through a step by step approach to find the areas of weakness and with easy to apply, natural solutions I was able to start my journey to healing."

—Wendy McElderry

"As an older late 30 something new mama
I was concerned about my over health before
getting pregnant. Many friends were experiencing
morning sickness, fatigue, and constipation.
I didn't want to be one of those moms to not enjoy
my pregnancy. I followed the protocol to cleanse
my colon and entire body through
Dr LeAnne Deardeuff's recommendations and did
not experience—not one day—any symptoms of
morning sickness from beginning to end. We are
very grateful and now inspire other women to do
the same. Dr LeAnne has been the only one to tell
it to us straight about cleansing and toxins. You
really do need all the energy you can get!"

—Jennifer Hitchcock